Pub. 18.23

PROGRESS IN CLINICAL AND BIOLOGICAL RESEARCH

RECENT TITLES

Vol 53: **Cancer Among Black Populations,** Curtis Mettlin and Gerald P. Murphy, *Editors*

Vol 54: **Connective Tissue Research: Chemistry, Biology, and Physiology,** Zdenek Deyl and Milan Adam, *Editors*

Vol 55: **The Red Cell: Fifth Ann Arbor Conference,** George J. Brewer, *Editor*

Vol 56: **Erythrocyte Membranes 2: Recent Clinical and Experimental Advances,** Walter C. Kruckeberg, John W. Eaton, and George J. Brewer, *Editors*

Vol 57: **Progress in Cancer Control,** Curtis Mettlin and Gerald P. Murphy, *Editors*

Vol 58: **The Lymphocyte,** Kenneth W. Sell and William V. Miller, *Editors*

Vol 59: **Eleventh International Congress of Anatomy,** Enrique Acosta Vidrio, *Editor-in-Chief.* Published in 3 volumes:
  Part A: **Glial and Neuronal Cell Biology,** Sergey Fedoroff, *Editor*
  Part B: **Advances in the Morphology of Cells and Tissues,** Miguel A. Galina, *Editor*
  Part C: **Biological Rhythms in Structure and Function,** Heinz von Mayersbach, Lawrence E. Scheving, and John E. Pauly, *Editors*

Vol 60: **Advances in Hemoglobin Analysis,** Samir M. Hanash and George J. Brewer, *Editors*

Vol 61: **Nutrition and Child Health: Perspectives for the 1980s,** Reginald C. Tsang and Buford Lee Nichols, Jr., *Editors*

Vol 62: **Pathophysiological Effects of Endotoxins at the Cellular Level,** Jeannine A. Majde and Robert J. Person, *Editors*

Vol 63: **Membrane Transport and Neuroreceptors,** Dale Oxender, Arthur Blume, Ivan Diamond, and C. Fred Fox, *Editors*

Vol 64: **Bacteriophage Assembly,** Michael S. DuBow, *Editor*

Vol 65: **Apheresis: Development, Applications, and Collection Procedures,** C. Harold Mielke, Jr., *Editor*

Vol 66: **Control of Cellular Division and Development,** Dennis Cunningham, Eugene Goldwasser, James Watson, and C. Fred Fox, *Editors.* Published in 2 volumes.

Vol 67: **Nutrition in the 1980s: Constraints on Our Knowledge,** Nancy Selvey and Philip L. White, *Editors*

Vol 68: **The Role of Peptides and Amino Acids as Neurotransmitters,** J. Barry Lombardini and Alexander D. Kenny, *Editors*

Vol 69: **Twin Research 3, Proceedings of the Third International Congress on Twin Studies,** Luigi Gedda, Paolo Parisi, and Walter E. Nance, *Editors.* Published in 3 volumes:
  Part A: **Twin Biology and Multiple Pregnancy**
  Part B: **Intelligence, Personality, and Development**
  Part C: **Epidemiological and Clinical Studies**

Vol 70: **Reproductive Immunology,** Norbert Gleicher, *Editor*

Vol 71: **Psychopharmacology of Clonidine,** Harbans Lal and Stuart Fielding, *Editors*

Vol 72: **Hemophilia and Hemostasis,** Doris Ménaché, D. MacN. Surgenor, and Harlan D. Anderson, *Editors*

Vol 73:   **Membrane Biophysics: Structure and Function in Epithelia,** Mumtaz A. Dinno and
          Arthur B. Callahan, *Editors*

Vol 74:   **Physiopathology of Endocrine Diseases and Mechanisms of Hormone Action,**
          Roberto J. Soto, Alejandro De Nicola, and Jorge Blaquier, *Editors*

Vol 75:   **The Prostatic Cell: Structure and Function,** Gerald P. Murphy, Avery A. Sandberg,
          and James P. Karr, *Editors*. Published in 2 volumes:
              Part A: **Morphologic, Secretory, and Biochemical Aspects**
              Part B: **Prolactin, Carcinogenesis, and Clinical Aspects**

Vol 76:   **Troubling Problems in Medical Ethics: The Third Volume in a Series on Ethics,
          Humanism, and Medicine,** Marc D. Basson, Rachel E. Lipson, and Doreen L.
          Ganos, *Editors*

Vol 77:   **Nutrition in Health and Disease and International Development: Symposia From the
          XII International Congress of Nutrition,** Alfred E. Harper and George K. Davis,
          Editors

Vol 78:   **Female Incontinence,** Norman R. Zinner and Arthur M. Sterling, *Editors*

See pages 285–286 for previous titles in this series.

TROUBLING PROBLEMS IN MEDICAL ETHICS

**The Third Volume in a Series on
Ethics, Humanism, and Medicine**

TROUBLING PROBLEMS IN MEDICAL ETHICS

The Third Volume in a Series on Ethics, Humanism, and Medicine

Proceedings of the 1980 and 1981 Conferences on
Ethics, Humanism, and Medicine at the
University of Michigan, Ann Arbor

Editors
MARC D. BASSON
RACHEL E. LIPSON
DOREEN L. GANOS

ALAN R. LISS, INC., NEW YORK

Address all Inquiries to the Publisher
Alan R. Liss, Inc., 150 Fifth Avenue, New York, NY 10011

Copyright © 1981 Alan R. Liss, Inc.

Printed in the United States of America.

Library of Congress Cataloging in Publication Data

Main entry under title:

Troubling problems in medical ethics.

    (Progress in clinical and biological research; 76)
    Includes bibliographical references and index.
    1. Medical ethics–Congresses. 2. Medical ethics–Case studies–Congresses. I. Basson, Marc D. II. Lipson, Rachel E. III. Ganos, Doreen L. IV. Title. V. Series. [DNLM: Ethics, Medical–United States–Congresses. W1 PR668E v. 78/ W 50 C7415 1980-81t]
R724.C618   174'.2   81-20723
ISBN 0-8451-0076-9

Contents

Contributors ix
About the Authors xi
Preface
  Marc D. Basson xvii
Sixth Conference
  Marc D. Basson: Acting With Uncertainty 3
  Affirmative Action in Medical School Admissions
    Doreen L. Ganos: Introduction 9
    Case for Discussion 13
    Carl Cohen: Affirmative Action in Medical School Admissions . . 17
    H. Jack Geiger: Affirmative Action in Medical School
      Admissions 39
    Doreen L. Ganos: Discussion Summary 47
  Drug Testing in Prisons
    Laurie Winkelman: Introduction 49
    Case for Discussion 53
    Marx Wartofsky: The Prisoners' Dilemma: Drug Testing in
      Prisons and the Violation of Human Rights 57
    Robert J. Levine: Drug Testing in Prisons 73
    Pat Duffy, Jr.: Drug Testing in Prisons: The View
      From Inside 79
    Laurie Winkelman: Discussion Summary 91
  Treating Children Without Parental Consent
    Rachel E. Lipson: Introduction 95
    Case for Discussion 97
    Robert A. Burt: Treating Children Without Parental Consent 101
    Arnold S. Relman: Treating Children Without Parental Consent . 109
    Rachel E. Lipson: Discussion Summary 115
  The Decision to Resuscitate—Slowly
    Marc D. Basson: Introduction 117
    Case for Discussion 119
    Martin Benjamin: Patient Autonomy and the Decision
      to Resuscitate "Without Undue Haste" 123
    David R. Dantzker: The Decision to Resuscitate—Slowly 131
    Marc D. Basson: Discussion Summary 141

Seventh Conference

Marc D. Basson: Approaches to Ethics 145

Competence and the Right to Refuse Treatment

Rachel E. Lipson: Introduction 151

Case for Discussion 153

Edward B. Goldman: Competency and the Right to Refuse
Treatment: Who's in Charge? 157

Robert L. Sadoff: Competency and the Right to
Refuse Treatment 169

Marc D. Basson: Discussion Summary 177

When Doctor and Nurse Disagree

Daria Chapelsky: Introduction 179

Case for Discussion 183

Mila Ann Aroskar: When Doctor and Nurse Disagree: An
Interface of Politics and Ethics 187

Robert H. Bartlett: When Doctor and Nurse Disagree 193

Daria Chapelsky: Discussion Summary 203

Doctor Draft: Redistributing Physicians

Barbara Weil: Introduction 207

Case for Discussion 209

Lance K. Stell: Stop the Draft: Why Compulsory
Redistribution of Physicians Would be Wrong 213

Joanne E. Lukomnik: Redistributing Physician Services:
Some Ethical Issues 227

Barbara Weil: Discussion Summary 235

The Right to Privacy When Lives Are at Stake

Marc D. Basson: Introduction 239

Case for Discussion 241

Arthur L. Caplan: The Right to Privacy When Lives
Are at Stake 245

Gerald D. Abrams: The Right to Privacy When Lives
Are at Stake 257

Marc D. Basson: Discussion Summary 269

References 273

Index 281

Contributors

Gerald D. Abrams, M.D. [257]
Department of Pathology, M4237 Med Sci I, Box 045, University of Michigan, Ann Arbor, Michigan 48109

Mila Ann Aroskar, R.N., Ed.D. [187]
University of Minnesota School of Public Health, 1360 Mayo Memorial Building, 420 Delaware Street S.E., Minneapolis, Minnesota 55455

Robert H. Bartlett, M.D. [193]
Department of Surgery, School of Medicine, University of Michigan, Ann Arbor, Michigan 48109

Marc D. Basson, M.D [xvii, 3, 13, 53, 97, 117, 119, 141, 145, 153, 177, 183, 209, 239, 241, 269]
Department of Surgery, Columbia Presbyterian Medical Center, West 168th Street, New York, New York 10032

Martin Benjamin, Ph.D. [123]
Department of Philosophy, Michigan State University, East Lansing, Michigan 48824

Robert A. Burt, J.D. [101]
Yale Law School, New Haven, Connecticut 06520

Arthur L. Caplan, Ph.D. [245]
The Hastings Institute for Society, Ethics and Life Sciences, 360 Broadway, Hastings on Hudson, New York 10706

Daria Chapelsky [179, 183, 203]
Committee on Ethics, Humanism, and Medicine, Inteflex, East Quad, University of Michigan, Ann Arbor, Michigan 48109

Carl Cohen, Ph.D. [17]
Department of Philosophy, Residential College, University of Michigan, Ann Arbor, Michigan 48109

David R. Dantzker, M.D. [131]
Department of Internal Medicine, S11303 Hospital, University of Michigan Medical School, Ann Arbor, Michigan 48109

Pat Duffy, Jr. [79]
c/o Mr. L.C. Utess, Director, Resident Services, Jackson State Prison, 4000 Cooper Street, Jackson, Michigan 49201

The bold face numbers in brackets following contributors' names indicate the opening page numbers of their papers.

Doreen L. Ganos, B.S. [9, 47]
  1015 East Ann Street, Apartment 2C, Ann Arbor, Michigan 48104
H. Jack Geiger, M.D. [39]
  School of Biomedical Education, City College of New York, 138th Street and
  Convent Avenue, New York, New York 10031
Edward B. Goldman, J.D. [157]
  Hospital Attorney's Office, University Hospital, 1405 East Ann Street, Ann
  Arbor, Michigan 48109
Robert J. Levine, M.D. [73]
  Department of Internal Medicine, Room C-407 SHM, Yale University, 333
  Cedar Street, New Haven, Connecticut 06510
Rachel E. Lipson, A.B. [13, 95, 97, 115, 151]
  1080 Island Drive Court, Apartment 105, Ann Arbor, Michigan 48105
Joanne Lukomnik, M.D. [227]
  Department of Community Medicine at the Sophie Davis School of Biomedical
  Education of the City College of New York, 138th St. and Convent Avenue,
  New York, New York 10031
Arnold S. Relman, M.D. [109]
  Editor, The New England Journal of Medicine, 10 Shattuck Street, Boston,
  Massachusetts 02115
Robert L. Sadoff, M.D. [169]
  Suite 326, The Benjamin Fox Pavilion, Jenkintown, Pennsylvania 19046
Lance K. Stell, Ph.D. [213]
  Department of Philosophy, Davidson College, Davidson, North Carolina 28036
Marx Wartofsky, Ph.D. [57]
  Department of Philosophy, Boston University, 745 Commonwealth Avenue,
  Boston, Massachusetts 02215
Barbara Weil [207, 209, 235]
  Committee on Ethics, Humanism, and Medicine, Inteflex, East Quad,
  University of Michigan, Ann Arbor, Michigan 48109
Laurie Winkelman [49, 53, 91, 241]
  Committee on Ethics, Humanism, and Medicine, Inteflex, East Quad,
  University of Michigan, Ann Arbor, Michigan 48109

ABOUT THE AUTHORS

Gerald Abrams is currently Professor of Pathology at the
University of Michigan and has been a member of the faculty
for many years. In addition to his work in pathology, Dr.
Abrams has had a longstanding commitment to the teaching of
medical ethics. He was instrumental in the establishment
and growth of the University of Michigan Medical School's
original Program in Health and Human Values and has subsequently been an enthusiastic participant in that medical
school's lecture series on the medical humanities.

Mila Aroskar is Associate Professor of Public Health Nursing
at the University of Minnesota School of Public Health. She
also has an extensive background in clinical nursing and has
frequently been called upon as an advisor on both clinical
and educational problems of nursing ethics. She spent
a year at Harvard's Interfaculty Program in Medical Ethics,
has coedited an anthology entitled "Ethical Dilemmas in
Nursing Practice" with Anne Davis, and has written extensively
on problems in nursing ethics.

Robert Bartlett received his MD from the University of
Michigan, trained in general and thoracic surgery at the
Peter Bent Brigham Hospital in Boston and then spent several
years on the faculty of the University of California before
returning to the University of Michigan in 1980 as Professor
of General and Thoracic Surgery. As Director of the Surgical
Intensive Care Unit at University Hospital and of the Department of Surgery's resident training program, he has had
extensive practical experiences of cases of physician-
nurse disagreement and combines this experience with a

longstanding interest in and sensitivity to the concerns of medical ethics.

Marc D. Basson founded the Committee on Ethics, Humanism and Medicine in 1978 and served as its director though 1981, when the seventh of these conferences was held. He received his AB from the University of Michigan in "Philosophy of Medicine" and subsequently did a student internship at the Institute for Society, Ethics and the Life Sciences. In addition to editing previous volumes of CEHM proceedings, he has written on medical ethics for several journals. Having graduated from the University of Michigan Medical School, he is currently a house officer in the Department of Surgery at the Columbia Presbyterian Medical Center.

Martin Benjamin is Professor of Philosophy at Michigan State University. He was Assistant Coordinator of the Medical Humanities Program from 1979-80 and has taught in Michigan State's two medical colleges. For over six years he has participated in and helped organize a series of monthly case conferences on ethical issues in Lansing hospitals. Among his written works are a number of papers on ethics and medicine (in particular on problems relating to death) and a book (co-authored with Joy Curtis) on "Ethics in Nursing."

Robert Burt is currently Professor of Law at Yale University and Co-Chairman of the Program in Law and Medicine at Yale Law School. He is a fellow of the Hastings Institute for Society, Ethics and the Life Sciences and has written extensively on proxy consent and children's rights.

Arthur Caplan is Associate for the Humanities at the Hastings Institute for Society, Ethics and the Life Sciences as well as Associate for Social Medicine in the Department of Medicine at the Columbia University College of Physicians and Surgeons. His major areas of interest include history and philosophy of the life sciences, philosophy of science and ethical issues in science and medicine. He has written and spoken extensively on a vast range of topics throughout these areas and has recently become interested in a theoretical analysis of the right to privacy.

Daria Chapelsky is a nursing student at the University of Michigan. An active member of the Committee on Ethics, Humanism and Medicine, she coordinates the Committee's series of Nursing Brown Bag Luncheons as well as working on the Committee's publicity efforts.

Carl Cohen is Professor of Philosophy at the Residential
College of the University of Michigan. He has written
extensively on the philosophical ramifications of diverse
public policy issues including medical experimentation on
human subjects, privacy, recombinant DNA technology, and
affirmative action. He serves as a member of the Human
Subject Review Committee of the University of Michigan
Medical School and has been Chairman of the American Civil
Liberties Union of Michigan and a member of the National
Board of Directors of the ACLU.

David Dantzker is an Associate Professor of Medicine at
the University of Michigan Medical School. He has extensive
experience with respiratory intensive care unit medicine and
has long been interested in medical ethics.

Pat Duffy is an inmate at Jackson State Prison in Jackson,
Michigan and has participated in many of the studies performed on prisoners in that institution by the pharmaceutical
industry.

Doreen L. Ganos received her BS in Biomedical Sciences from
the University of Michigan and is currently a third year
medical student there. She has been a member of the Committee
on Ethics, Humanism and Medicine from its founding in 1978,
and currently serves as Director for Publicity and Registration and Chief Financial Officer for the Committee.

H. Jack Geiger is Arthur C. Logan Professor of Community
Medicine and Director of the Program in Health, Medicine and
Society at the School of Biomedical Education of the City
College of New York. He serves on the Governing Council of
the American Public Health Association and was a consultant
for policy research on medically underserved areas for the
National Center for Health Services Research of the Department
of Health, Education and Welfare. He has written on issues
of public health, medical ethics, and medical education.

Edward B. Goldman is the attorney for health care at the
University of Michigan and a lecturer at the University of
Michigan Law School. In addition to his practical exper-
ience with many cases of questionably competent patients at
University Hospital, Mr. Goldman's background includes the
teaching of several seminars on psychiatry and the law, a

lecture series on medical law at the University of Michigan
Medical School, and long and enthusiastic advice and support
to the Committee on Ethics, Humanism and Medicine.

Robert Levine is currently Professor of Medicine and Lecturer
in Pharmacology at Yale. He has long been active in matters
of public policy, medical law, and medical ethics. He is the
founding editor of "IRB: A Review of Human Subjects Research,"
chairs the Human Investigation Committee at Yale which
reviews all clinical research, and is a panelist for the
FDA's quarterly workshops on Institutional Review Boards. He
also served on the National Committee for the Protection of
Human Subjects of Biomedical and Behavioral Research. He
has written and spoken widely on human experimentation and
informed consent.

Rachel Lipson is a student at the Univeristy of Michigan
Medical School. She has been working on the Committee on
Ethics, Humanism and Medicine since its inception in 1978
and is currently the Committee's Program Director.

Joanne Lukomnik was Medical Director of the National Health
Service Corps at the time she delivered this paper and has
recently joined the Department of Community Medicine at the
Sophie Davis School of Biomedical Education of the City
College of New York. She has had a longstanding interest in
the community health center movement and in women's health
issues.

Arnold Relman's interest in ethics dates back to an undergraduate major in philosophy. His more recent activities
include editing the New England Journal of Medicine, serving
on the Editorial Advisory Board of "Science" and holding a
professorship at Harvard Medical School. He has recently
been appointed to the Board of Directors for the Hastings
Institute for Society, Ethics and the Life Sciences. He has
written extensively in the New England Journal and elsewhere
on matters of medical ethics and public policy.

Robert Sadoff is Professor of Psychiatry at the University
of Pennsylvania and a lecturer at the Villanova University
School of Law. He brings to the topic of patient competence
to refuse treatment both a long clinical experience with
problems of this sort and major academic and research interests
at the interface between psychiatry and the law.

Lance Stell is Associate Professor of Philosophy at Davidson College, where he teaches an undergraduate course in medical ethics. His major professional interests involve social and economic philosophy, with particular reference to the conflict between social justice and individual liberties.

Marx Wartofsky is Professor of Philosophy and previously was chairman of the Department of Philosophy at Boston University. He serves on the editorial committee of the Journal of Medicine and Philosophy and as the Director of the Boston Colloquium for the Philosophy of Science, among other activities. He is affiliated with the American Philosophical Association, the American Association for the Advancement of Science, the Society for Health and Human Values and the American Civil Liberties Union. He has written a great deal on philosophy of science and political philosophy.

Barbarba Weil is an undergraduate economics major at the University of Michigan who has been with the Committee on Ethics, Humanism and Medicine for two years. She currently serves as Assistant Director of Publicity and Assistant Director for Finance.

Laurie Winkelman is a student at the University of Michigan Medical School. She has been a member of the Committee on Ethics, Humanism and Medicine for the last two years and is currently the Committee's Assistant Program Director.

PREFACE

Marc D. Basson
Director, CEHM
University of Michigan
Ann Arbor, Michigan

The Committee on Ethics, Humanism and Medicine (CEHM)
has grown steadily since it was founded in 1978. With what
we take to be pardonable pride, we believe it unique among
student organizations in terms of the range and sophistication
of activities it sponsors. These currently include regular
Ethics Grand Rounds at the Ann Arbor Veterans Administration
Hospital, a series of brown bag luncheons at the University
of Michigan School of Nursing, and many other seminars at
Michigan's Medical School and College of Literature, Science
and the Arts. In addition to these local activities, aimed
primarily at increasing the ethical sophistication of the
University community, CEHM organizes and directs two major
conferences each year on issues in medical ethics. The
present volume represents the proceedings of the sixth and
seventh of these conferences, held during the 1980-81
academic year. (Proceedings of the first five conferences
have already been published in two earlier volumes in this
series entitled "Ethics, Humanism and Medicine" and "Rights
and Responsibilities in Modern Medicine.")

These conferences are interdisciplinary in nature, with
speakers and participants from such fields as medicine,
nursing, public health, philosophy, religion, and law.
Conference registration generally ranges between 250 and
400, including faculty and students from the University of
Michigan and other midwestern universities as well as practicing
health care professionals, attorneys, philosophers, and other
interested lay persons. Topics for discussion at each
conference are selected by the Committee from the votes and
suggestions of participants at previous conferences, and

from issues of current concern. We aim to provoke and
"raise consciousness" but also to educate participants about
the issues in question.

The major thrust of these conferences is toward demon-
strating the application to medical issues of techniques of
rational ethical analysis and argument. The conferences are
uniquely structured to facilitate this goal. Each topic is
introduced by two speakers from different disciplines (generally one a clinician and one a non-clinician) who illustrate
their own approaches to the topic. Then participants divide
into prearranged discussion groups of ten to twelve people.
There, they are given a case to discuss and are charged with
answering on their own (and preferably unanimously) a
series of questions about the ethical issues implicit in the
situation described. The emphasis is on logical analysis
rather than "correct" answers. The results of these discussions are summarized at the end of each topic's proceedings
so that the reader may compare his moral reasoning and
intuitions with those of the participants.

Organizing such conferences is no small task for a
group of full-time students, and great credit is due to all
the students who worked on CEHM projects and to those non-
students who have supported the CEHM effort. In order
to keep the price of this volume within manageable limits,
we can only mention some of those who helped.

My co-editors, Rachel Lipson and Doreen Ganos, have
served ably as Directors for Program and for Publicity and
Registration respectively, shouldering most of the work load
when the demands of clinical rotations distracted me from
CEHM. Barbara Weil, Assistant Publicity Director, coordinated
much of the effort that led to record attendances at these
conferences and produced an exceptionally rich and hetero-
genous group of participants. She also served as Assistant
Financial Director. Sandeep Shekar acted as Assistant
Registration Director and Laurie Winkelman as Assistant
Program Director. Daria Chapelsky contributed greatly to
our publicity efforts as well as coordinating our liaison
with the School of Nursing and organizing the CEHM Nursing
Ethics Brown Bag Luncheons which involved significant numbers
of nursing personnel in our activities for the first time
this year.

Elena Booker, Phil Dutt, Mary Fox, Juanita Kus, Kathy

McPhee, Eric Shampaine, Monica Sircar, Anthony So, and Don
Weston all contributed significantly to the organization of
these conferences. Other workers included Chuck Alejos,
Denise Campbell, Robert Flora, Duane Gall, Russ Herschelmann,
Dominique Hoppe, Carol Kahn, Grace Lee, Paul Lee, Andy
Leifer, Loren Levy, Steve Manley, Steve McCornick, Douglas
Mossman, Kumar Nalluswami, Jonathan Oppenheimer, Greg Pamel,
Jill Preston, Don Robinson, Karen Salem, Paul Shabaz,
Anthony So, Don Stasie, Mary Swastek, Lori Wissman, and
Elaine Zielke.

Several of the students listed above also participated
in the researching of cases for discussion and the writing
of supporting material for this volume, as is indicated
throughout these proceedings.

Our enthusiastic thanks are also due to many University
faculty and staff without whose guidance, encouragement and
support these conferences could never have occurred. To
Professor Carl Cohen, who first stimulated my own interest
in philosophy and who has been an enthusiastic supporter of
my own professional growth in medical ethics for the last
six years, to whom I have always been able to turn for
suggestions and advice since founding CEHM, I am deeply
grateful. University Hospital Attorney Edward Goldman has
likewise been a never-ending source of ideas, advice and
encouragement. Dr. Marcia Liepman has been a valuable
source for technical medical details in addition to providing close readings and commentaries on several of the
discussion cases as we developed them. Meredith Eiker has
been a valuable resource person for information on problems
of public policy and health care delivery as well as providing
continual and crucial support for the VA Hospital Ethics
Grand Rounds that have provided us with valuable links to
that institution. Dr. Gerald Abrams, Dr. Robert Bartlett,
Dr. Ronald Bishop, Dr. David Dantzker, Dr. Terence Davies,
Dr. Carolyne Davis, Dr. Errol Erlandson, Professor Nancy
Prince, and Dr. Jane Schultz have all been most helpful at
many points along the way to developing these conferences.

Special thanks are also due to Susan Anker, Alice
Cohen, Helen Ferran, Shirley Martin, Aurelia Navarro, and
Ann Zinn, who have volunteered much of their time in coping
with the barrage of administrative paperwork and correspond-
ence necessary for organizing these conferences and register-
ing hundreds of participants. We are additionally grateful

to Aurelia Navarro for her fine work in transcribing speakers'
presentations and doing other typing for this volume.

Support for these conferences has been provided by the
College of Literature, Science and the Arts, The Collegiate
Institute for Values and Science, Dr Carolyne Davis, the
Department of Family Practice, the Integrated Premedical-
Medical Program, Dr. Charles G. Overberger, the Rackham
School of Graduate Studies, the Law School, the Medical
School, the School of Nursing, the School of Pharmacy, and
the School of Public Health, all of the University of Michigan.

As the preparation of this volume represents the conclusion
of my own tenure with the Committee, I add my personal
gratitude to that of the Committee for the support of all
these people and institutions and in particular for the
students who have sacrificed studying and leisure time to
create the organization that CEHM has become. If we have
succeeding in teaching even a few conference participants
what it means to reason logically about ethical questions,
I will count all our effort not wasted, for it will be
multiplied by all the years each of those participants lives
to put his learnings into practice. I hope that we have
additionally added somewhat to the general level of ethical
sophistication in the University of Michigan medical community and trust that the Committee will live long and prosper
in this milieu.

Sixth Conference on
Ethics, Humanism, and Medicine
November 8, 1980

**Troubling Problems in Medical Ethics: The Third
Volume in a Series on Ethics, Humanism, and Medicine: 3–8
© 1981 Alan R. Liss, Inc., 150 Fifth Ave., New York, NY 10011**

INTRODUCTION TO THE SIXTH CONFERENCE: ACTING WITH UNCERTAINTY

Marc D. Basson
Director, CEHM
University of Michigan Medical School
Ann Arbor, Michigan

Good morning and welcome to the Sixth Conference on
Ethics, Humanism, and Medicine.

You will hear several distinguished and thoughtful
speakers today, each sharing with you his approach to particular problems in medical ethics. But when all the papers
have been presented we will ask you to make a series of
decisions about the cases in your program.

This will not be an easy task. Many of you may feel
that you lack sufficient medical knowledge or ethical sophistication. Yet this is as it should be if these exercises are
to simulate the real world. For we must all too often in
medicine arrive at answers before we clearly understand the
questions, in situations which render us acutely conscious of
how little we know and how unsure we are of our beliefs.

A certain arrogance is required for making decisions
under such circumstances, a readiness to believe in oneself
and one's best guess when lives are at stake, even while
acknowledging the possibility of error. The lack of such
self-confidence paralyzes. James Childress, for example,
rejects ethical decision-making based on cost-benefit analysis
because of the chance of error. "God may be a utilitarian,
but we cannot be," notes Childress (1970). "We simply lack
the capacity to predict very accurately the consequences" of
our decisions. Too much belief in one's infallibility, on
the other hand, may create a paternalistic monster. One
surgeon advises medical students that "the request for
permission would be presented...in such a way that he feels

he has no option to refuse....Despite all efforts to the contrary there will still be a few patients who defy rational management and refuse to cooperate. Restraint is occasionally necessary for the confused and irrational adult." (Fisher, 1977). The zone between timidity and overconfidence is so narrow that our decision-making becomes fraught with ambivalence and guilt. "What right has the doctor to play God?" asks the magazine article. "Who shall decide?" cries the bioethics text.

I contend that these are the wrong questions. I would like to show you why these questions are poor and then to replace them with some better questions which I will leave equally unanswered. Issues of medical ethics are difficult, and there are rarely satisfactory answers. It is understandable that those once our patients and now consumers of our health care demand a voice in such decisions, if not the right to decide all by themselves. But it would be horribly wrong for us to allow patients to decide alone how we ought to treat them. The physician who pulls a plug that he believes ought to remain connected because a patient or a court orders disconnection is, I contend, as morally responsible for his act as the doctors who supervised studies in slow death in Nazi concentration camps because of orders from above. The doctor <u>must</u> decide, even if his decision is simply that either option is acceptable to him and that he will therefore abide by the patient's wishes.

Think, if this bothers you, of the medical school professor who goes back to the Admissions Office after rounds to choose among applicants to medical school. With a stroke of his pen or a single sarcastic word he may reject or accept an applicant, and thus dramatically alter not only the applicant's life, but also the lives of his family and of the patients the candidate might have served. These are hard choices, and have consequences potentially as serious as any in medicine. Yet we do not challenge the admissions officer with: "Who are you to make such decisions?" He makes them because somebody must and he has been appointed. Instead, better questions to ask of him are, "How do you make these decisions? How ought you to make them? What should you consider?"

Similarly, a better question to ask of physician choices in patient treatment is, "What ought the physician consider in his decision?" Potentially relevant factors include the interests of the patient, those of his family or friends, and those of society. I believe that the interests of the patient's family should never justify an action against the patient's own interests and that the good of society should contravene the patient's own good only because of considerations of scarce resources or threatened harm by the patient to others. Others will disagree, and I leave this for you to discuss.

The patient's own interests are much more problematic for me. The doctor must separate what he believes is good for the patient from what the patient actually wants or would want if he could be asked. There is often a great temptation to override a patient's decision for his own good, because the patient knows not what he does. Paternalism is the doctrine that one may violate a person's autonomy to save him from himself. It has a venerable tradition in medical ethics, dating back to the Hippocratic doctors who swore to "come for the benefit of the sick" and "to keep them from harm" regardless of the irrational desires of their patients.

But paternalism is coming under attack today. It is clear, for instance, that physicians as a group are significantly biased toward aggressive medical therapy as compared to the rest of the population (Aring, 1968; Feifel, et al., 1967). They are much more likely to want their tumors excised, their diseases treated, their lungs ventilated, even when they know that the chance of cure is nil and the chance of significant palliation minimal. What is more, they want this for their patients as well, and many are prepared to declare patients irrational or incompetent if they do not wish these things. On the contrary, we are now learning that the patient who refuses therapy or diagnostic testing may be perfectly rational, but might simply prefer not to know that she has untreatable cancer or might prefer to die now rather than later. Patient preferences for "death with dignity" or for life at all costs represent differences in values and not errors in logic. I contend that a patient may be declared incompetent if he is insane or incapable of appreciating the facts he needs to make a decision, but not if he disagrees about the importance of such facts.

In fact, competent patients have been held to have a legal "right to act foolishly" (In re Yetter, 1973), and many philosophers believe this to be a moral right as well. This right of foolish action is said to be limited only by the demonstration of clear errors in information or reasoning on

the part of the patient or by emergencies which make it
impossible to evaluate the patient's mental status. (In
emergencies, an old doctrine urges us to err on the side of
life and reversibility.) It has also been noted that while
the patient has a right to act foolishly, the doctor has no
obligation to follow that lead. A patient may refuse surgery,
but may not demand poison.

It is sometimes argued that there are circumstances in
which a patient's request must be honored, but in which he
need not be given a chance to make such a request. The
doctor in our fourth case today, for instance, argues that to
consult with the patient about euthanasia would cause mental
anguish not worth the bit of life she has left. Placebo
treatment is another example of circumstances preventing
discussion with the patient. The ethical validity of such
practices is debatable. I think that if nothing else, there
is certainly a prima facie case for consulting with all
competent patients before administering or withdrawing
treatment. The burden of proof (it seems to me) is on those
who propose to avoid such discussion.

Matters become even more difficult when the patient is
either unable to communicate or of questionable competence.
Non-communicative patients (either unconscious or locked-in
after a stroke) must have decisions made for them by proxy.
There are two theories of proxy consent, based on the distinction between interests and desires and thus differing on
which of these the patient's proxy ought to honor for her.
If people have a right to act foolishly, then perhaps these
desires ought to be honored by proxy as well.

Of course it is often hard to determine how a patient
would act if only he were conscious, pain-free, and rational
when he is none of these. The notion of using the patient's
next of kin as his proxy has some roots in the old idea that
a child or a deceased person's corpse is the property of his
family. Fortuitously, the family is also (or so it has been
said) the most likely to understand the patient's desires and
to have his best interests at heart. But this is not always
the case, and particularly now that we have learned to distinguish desire from interest many have suggested that the
proxy should not automatically revert to the next of kin. A
bill in the Michigan legislature proposes that the patient be
allowed to designate his own proxy in advance. Others have
suggested that if this is impossible, the physician ought to

go to court and get a guardian appointed or that the doctor ought to take it upon himself to weigh all the evidence and then decide.

Patients who can communicate their desires at least imperfectly but who are of questionable competence pose special problems. Children, the senile, and the mentally disturbed are examples of such patients. Many have argued that the expressed wishes of these people ought to be considered as evidence of what they would wish if they were in fact competent. This is not perfect evidence, for surely we all have seen children refusing an injection and forced it upon them, reasoning that if only they were older they would understand and accept. But it does seem helpful in decision-making. The problems arise when we ask such a patient for his consent to bolster our case and he then refuses. It is much more difficult emotionally to perform a procedure on an unwilling patient than on an unknowing one. Some have argued that the physician's emotional reaction in such cases stems from a moral intuition that even such patients ought to have some say in their management, while others take the position that our disquiet only reflects the similarity of such cases to forcing treatment on clearly competent patients. Like the other issues I have raised, I leave this one unresolved.

I would like to leave you with quotations from two of this century's great humanists. The first is by Dr. Oliver Cope, a noted surgeon from Harvard Medical School and Massachusetts General Hospital and a distinguished student of the process and goals of medical education. "The art of medicine," Dr. Cope explains, "is the ability to make the right decisions on inadequate evidence." (Cope, 1968) This holds for ethical decisions in medicine as well as scientific, and the possibility and consequences of error are awesome. Perhaps my second quote provides the answer, for which I am indebted to a paper by James Rachels. He cites a Peanuts cartoon in which Lucy muses, "Are there more bad people in the world or are there more good people?" "Who is to say?" Charlie Brown responds. "Who is to say who is bad or who is good?" Lucy has the answer: "I will," she says. This is my final message to you. The decisions are hard, but they must be made and you must make them. So clench your teeth on the proverbial bullet and accept what must be done. Be thoughtful but confident, for the alternative is paralysis.

Thank you for listening. I hope that the conference is both enjoyable and instructive for you.

REFERENCES

Aring CD (1968). Intimations of mortality: An appreciation
    of death and dying. Ann Int Med 69(July):139.
Childress JF (1970). Who shall live when not all can live?
    Soundings 43(4):339.
Cope O (1968). "Man, Mind and Medicine: The Doctor's
    Education." Philadelphia: JB Lippincott Company.
Feifel H, Hanson S. Jones R, Edwards E (1967). Physicians
    consider death. Proc 75th Annual Convention, American
    Psychological Assoc, p.201.
Fisher JC (1977). "Clinical Procedures." Baltimore:
    Williams and Wilkins.
Rachels J (1980). Can ethics provide answers? Hastings
    Center Report 10(3):32.
In re Appointment of a Guardian for the Person of Maida
    Yetter, Docket No. 1973-533 (Pa Ct of Common Pleas,
    Northampton Co. Orphans' Ct, June 6, 1973).

**Troubling Problems in Medical Ethics: The Third
Volume in a Series on Ethics, Humanism, and Medicine: 9–11
© 1981 Alan R. Liss, Inc., 150 Fifth Ave., New York, NY 10011**

INTRODUCTION: AFFIRMATIVE ACTION IN MEDICAL SCHOOL ADMISSIONS

Doreen L. Ganos
Director for Publicity and Registration
CEHM
University of Michigan
Ann Arbor, Michigan

Affirmative action in medical school admissions has been
stirring up controversy since the first programs began. The
dilemma at the heart of this controversy is that affirmative
action programs are usually designed not only to prevent
future discrimination but also to compensate for the effects
of past injustices, generally by offering preferential
treatment to the group previously discriminated against.
These programs therefore bring two basic moral principles
into conflict, that of "compensatory justice" and that of
"formal equality" which says that "equals must be treated
equally and unequals unequally." (Beauchamp, 1975)   This
often gives rise to cries of "reverse discrimination," meaning
"an action or a practice [that] discriminates against an
individual or a group on the basis of some normally irrelevant
criterion (such as race, sex, or ethnic origin) because
preference is being given to members of previously discriminated against groups." (Mappes & Zembaty, 1977) The Allan
Bakke case discussed in Professor Cohen's paper is a famous
example of this. Such cases pose complex ethical problems.
In addition to the basic principles already cited, one must
consider such other difficult questions as what role(s) a
medical school should play in the social order, and whether
equal treatment is possible without compensation for past
discrimination. The complexity of these issues may readily
lead to different conclusions even after careful study, as
evidenced by the speakers' disagreement.

Professor Cohen begins his paper by persuasively presenting four major arguments against the use of racial or
ethnic categories as a basis for preferential admissions

programs. First, he claims that such procedures are morally wrong because they often do not provide the compensatory relief for which they are intended, instead allotting rewards to undeserving individuals. Second, Professor Cohen points out that such programs blatantly violate the Civil Rights Act of 1964. Third, he notes that they are unconstitutional as well, since they violate the equal protection of the laws clause in the Fourteenth Amendment. Fourth, he warns that programs of racial preference are unwise, because they may increase inter-racial tensions and stereotype all members of preferred minorities as inferior and requiring special treatment. Professor Cohen goes on to explain the reasoning behind the complicated Bakke decision and the impact of this ruling, which allows only very limited considerations of race. Lastly, with an eye to his opening arguments, Cohen suggests that even this limited use might well be wisely forsworn.

In direct opposition, Dr. Geiger presents a strong argument in favor of using racial preferences in medical school admissions, concentrating on the social context in which these decisions are made. He considers two questions: one, are the current criteria for admission equitable or even relevant, and two, is admission to medical school a private good obtained on merit or a public good to be administered according to social needs? Discussing the first question, Geiger points out that such factors as economic pressures, lower quality school systems, and the lack of role models make the current scholastic criteria a "stacked deck" for people in the lower socioeconomic classes. Not only are such criteria as MCAT scores and grade point averages inequitable, he claims, but also they are largely irrelevant in choosing potentially good physicians so long as the applicant possesses a certain minimum level of intelligence and knowledge. In answering the second question, that of what role medical schools should play in society, Geiger declares that, because of the large proportion of public funds in medical school budgets, we should demand of medical schools that they fulfill societal goals in addition to their academic tasks. Geiger argues that medical schools should try to reduce inequities and to provide compensatory relief for access to medical school places as well as to health care, and that these goals can best be carried out through quotas (or perhaps stratified lotteries) that give preferential admittance on the basis of race and ethnicity.

REFERENCES

Beauchamp TL (1975). The justification of reverse discrim-
     ination. Reprinted in Mappes TA, Zembaty JS (eds)(1977).
     "Social Ethics: Morality and Social Policy." New York:
     McGraw-Hill, Inc.
Mappes TA, Zembaty JS (eds) (1977). "Social Ethics: Morality
     and Social Policy". New York: McGraw-Hill, Inc. p. 159.

**Troubling Problems in Medical Ethics: The Third
Volume in a Series on Ethics, Humanism, and Medicine: 13–16
© 1981 Alan R. Liss, Inc., 150 Fifth Ave., New York, NY 10011**

AFFIRMATIVE ACTION IN MEDICAL SCHOOL ADMISSIONS

CASE FOR DISCUSSION

You have just been appointed to the admissions committee at State Medical School to replace a fellow professor who suddenly had to retire for health reasons. It is nearing the end of summer and forty-eight candidates have been accepted for the fall freshman class. Two places, however, still remain open. The following eight applicants are being considered for these spots.

Bobby Chi is a 22 year old Asian American with a GPA of 3.7 and MCAT scores ranging from the 95th to the 98th percentile. Bobby comes from a middle class family and grew up in a suburban community. He received his undergraduate degree in Biomedical Engineering from Princeton, and although he has no experience working in a hospital or a medical setting, he says that he has always wanted to be a physician. He adds that he has learned "what medicine is about" in studying biomedical engineering. He was a member of the Princeton Engineering Society throughout his years in college.

Celia Jones is a 23 year old black woman with a GPA of 2.9 and MCAT scores ranging from the 70th to the 74th percentile. She grew up in the inner city and had to work her way through college because her family had no money. During her first three years at State College she worked both as a waitress and as a clerk in the hospital emergency room. She was forced to take a term off from college during her senior year because of lack of funds, but she worked during this time, and earned enough money to finish her degree in Developmental

Psychology last winter. She says that she wishes to
become a doctor so that she may return and help those
who live in the disadvantaged ghetto area where she
grew up. She was not involved in extracurricular
activities in college because of time constraints, but
she did spend a number of hours doing volunteer work at
a nearby nursing home.

Alex Miller is a 24 year old white man with a GPA of
3.5 and MCAT scores ranging from the 83rd to the 89th
percentile. He comes from a middle class family and he
grew up in New York City. He has a great interest in
political and social affairs, and describes himself as
having a "strong social conscience." Because of his
desire to help others, he spent two years in South
America with the Peace Corps after graduating from a
state university. After receiving his medical degree,
he plans to either return to the Peace Corps or to
practice some form of ghetto medicine, because he feels
these options will offer him the opportunity to help
the most people with the skills he has obtained.

Sharon Goldman is a 24 year old white woman with a GPA
of 3.8 and MCAT scores ranging from the 89th to the
95th percentile. She comes from an upper class family.
She has spent a great deal of time both during her
undergraduate and graduate years at Harvard doing
research in endocrinology. She explains that she became
interested in the subject during a physiology course
her freshman year and that she "just never lost interest".
She has multiple publications in the field, as well as
Bachelor's and Master's degrees. She has already been
accepted to the Ph.D. program in Physiology; however,
she just learned that if she is also accepted to the
medical school she can enter into a joint MD/PhD program.
She feels that with this background she will better be
able to pursue her research interests.

Leon Johnson is a 24 year old black man with a GPA of
3.6 and MCAT scores ranging from the 87th to the 91st
percentile. He grew up in the inner city, living with
his unwed mother who was on welfare. He won a scholarship to Howard University where he majored in Biology.
He did some research in biology while at Howard, and
has one publication in the field. He now states that
he wishes to become a plastic surgeon, and that he

hopes to make enough money so that his children will never know anything even close to the poverty in which he himself grew up. One interviewer suggested that perhaps if he worked as a physician in a ghetto neighborhood Leon would help many more children. Leon replied that he had worked his way out of the ghetto and he never planned to return.

Bill Tane is a 23 year old white man with a GPA of 3.0 and MCAT scores ranging from the 79th to the 83rd percentile. He grew up in rural Appalachia, where both his parents remain unemployed. He received a scholarship to a state college. He says he wants to be a neurosurgeon, because he especially enjoyed his classes in neurology. He also says that he hopes to return to his home community someday to help the people with whom he grew up.

Sherwin Williams is a 36 year old white man with a GPA of 3.9 and MCAT scores ranging from the 96th to the 98th percentile. He has a B.S. and a M.S. in engineering and owns a successful consulting firm. He had decided, however, that he is not happy in engineering because it is not "the right career" for him, and wishes to go into medicine because he fondly remembers working as an orderly at a local hospital while he was in high school. For the last three years, while taking basic premedical classes at night and earning a 4.0, he has also volunteered extensively at State University Hospital.

James Martin is a 23 year old black man with a GPA of 3.2 and MCAT scores ranging from the 79th to the 87th percetile. His father owns a chain of stores and he grew up in an upper class suburb. He attended Princeton and received his degree in Chemistry last spring. While in college he worked as a volunteer at the local hospital. He was involved in many college activities including the Glee Club, the volunteer service organization, and the student newspaper, but he did not achieve officership in any of these.

You and the rest of the admissions committee must now choose two of these candidates. You have been informed that for the past five years each incoming class has been made up of approximately 15% minority students in accordance with the University's non-binding affirmative action guidelines. If you accept two minority students at this point, then this year's class will have 14% minority members.

Which two students would you choose? Why? Would quotas have made your decision easier or harder? Would a quota have been an appropriate tool for decision making in this setting? What quotas (if any) would you use (e.g., blacks, minorities, people with deprived childhoods, people who would probably serve underprivileged areas)? If you did not use a quota but took such factors into account, how much ought they be weighted and why? What are the reasons for using quotas and affirmative action to modify straight merit selection in medical school admissions? How can these reasons be best served?

(Case prepared by Marc Basson, Rachel Lipson, Mary Fox, and Anthony So.)

Troubling Problems in Medical Ethics: The Third Volume in a Series on Ethics, Humanism, and Medicine: 17–38
© **1981 Alan R. Liss, Inc., 150 Fifth Ave., New York, NY 10011**

AFFIRMATIVE ACTION IN MEDICAL SCHOOL ADMISSIONS

Carl Cohen
Professor of Philosophy
Residential College
University of Michigan
Ann Arbor, Michigan

I divide my remarks into four short chapters. In the first I give a summary statement of my own judgments on the use of racial preference in medical school admissions. In the second I give an analysis of the substance of the Supreme Court decision in the wellknown Bakke case (1978). In the third I discuss some common criticisms of the outcome in Bakke. In the fourth I conclude with some general observations about medical school policies after Bakke.

CHAPTER I: ON RACIAL PREFERENCE AND AFFIRMATIVE ACTION

Preference given to some applicants for admission to professional school simply on the basis of race or ethnicity is wrong. I have presented the argument in support of this judgment at length elsewhere. (Cohen 1975, 1977, 1979a, 1979b) To provide a perspective on the analysis that follows, I recapitulate, very briefly, the reasons for this judgment.

The principle that all persons, without regard to race, religion, or sex, are entitled to the equal protection of the laws, is central in a just society. In practice this principle entails that racial and ethnic categories, as such, are not to be used in the application of the laws, or in the distribution of benefits under the law. The principle is a protection of each individual singly, and prohibits the invidious use of such categories in all public affairs.

The principle of equal protection does not forbid every use of racial categories. Where it can be shown that persons have been done an injustice because of their race, it is reasonable, of course, to recognize that racial cause, and to fashion appropriate remedies. Efforts to provide such remedies, under the name of affirmative action, have been widely undertaken by sensitive and honorable persons who seek to be fair. But in an effort to undo the results of past racial discrimination, many institutions have employed systems that are themselves discriminatory. Such discrimination, however well motivated, should be condemned. The conflict here is not between good guys and bad guys, but between differing views of how justice is to be pursued. On this there is, of course, much room for reasonable persons, all equally honorable, to disagree.

The issue is not whether to support or reject affirmative actions. (Cohen, 1979a) Affirmative action has a justifiably good name. It stands for honest steps taken either to eliminate discriminatory practices that were improper, or to provide corrective action where discriminatory practices had previously been employed. It is long past time for affirmative action so construed; a just society will take pride in it.

But what does affirmative action properly include? For many, affirmative action has come to mean the deliberate preference of some sheerly on the basis of their racial, sexual, or ethnic identification. Such flat discrimination, I contend, although sometimes called "affirmative action" and even sometimes identified with affirmative action, is wrongly confounded with appropriate compensatory relief. We may say, therefore, that affirmative action has healthy varieties (prophylactic as well as compensatory), and unhealthy varieties, in which attention is focused not upon the injury but upon group identification and the percentages (in medical school classes or elsewhere) with which ethnic groups are represented. It is with affirmative action of this second, unhealthy sort that the Bakke case was concerned. The upshot of that case was the prohibition of institutional preference because of race.

Four reasons may be given here, very summarily, for rejecting sheer racial preference in admissions.

1. Racial preference in medical school admissions is morally wrong. It takes from some for reasons that ought not to be considered, and gives to others for reasons that ought not to be considered. (Cohen, 1979a) It cannot be defended as compensatory, because it does not compensate many who have suffered the same injury, and does provide advantage for many who have not suffered injury. It is both underinclusive and overinclusive.

This objection to racial preference is not an objection to compensatory relief. Compensatory relief is often in order, after even a requirement of justice, common in law. To be just, however, compensatory relief must be designed to address the circumstances of persons who deserve relief because of the damage they have earlier suffered. It should provide relief in the light of the nature and degree of the injury suffered. It should be available to all those who have suffered injury of essentially the same kind, whatever their race or sex, and not be available to those who have not suffered that injury whatever their race or sex. Programs that give preference in admission simply on the basis of race or sex do not so tailor the remedy to the wrong. They attend, unjustly, to characteristics which, in themselves, are not injuries; we certainly ought not compensate people for being black, or brown, or female.

Of course it is true that many in one or another racial group have because of that identification borne certain sorts of burdens, and deserve compensation. But it is the burden for which relief is provided; we must therefore attend to whether or not individuals have been deprived. If the deprivation we seek to redress is academic, or economic, or familial, let us look to the question of who, among the applicants, have suffered that sort of deprivation. If we decide to compensate for such deprivations through preference in medical school admission--an instrument of possible but questionable appropriateness--let us give that compensatory preference to all who have borne that burden, regardless of their national origins, or color, or sex, or racial heritage. Racial preference, in sum, is entirely too blunt an instrument with which to approach the process of compensatory justice. (Cohen, 1975, 1977, 1979b)

2. Racial preference in medical school admissions
is legally wrong. It is, quite patently, a violation of
Federal law. Here is the law in question; it is Section
601 of the Civil Rights Act of 1964, as amended. It
reads, unambiguously, as follows:

> "No person in the United States shall,
> on the ground of race, color, or
> national origin, be excluded from
> participation in, be denied the
> benefits of, or be subjected to
> discrimination under any program
> or activity receiving Federal
> financial assistance."

This is plain, blunt language. It is repeated many
times, in many contexts, throughout the Civil Rights Act
of 1964--a Federal statute of which we are all justly
proud. One would have to be obtuse to deny that if any
individual is favored simply because of his race, for
goods that are in short supply and supported by Federal
funds (seats in a medical school. for example), some other
individual who loses out does so as a result of discrimination on the basis of race. That is flatly against the
law. Indeed, of the five justices of the United States
Supreme Court who found the special admissions program at
the University of California at Davis (in the Bakke case)
to be intolerable, four said that its illegality was perfectly plain; and all five said that it certainly was the
case that the Davis program violated the Civil Rights Act
of 1964.

3. Racial preference in medical school admissions
is constitutionally wrong. It violates the equal protection guarantee of the Fourteenth Amendment of the U.S.
Constitution which reads (in part) as follows: "nor shall
any State...deny to any person within its jurisdiction the
equal protection of the laws." Repeatedly the Supreme
Court has insisted that that guarantee is a protection of
individuals, that it applies to every and any single
person and not to groups. This aspect of the guarantee
has been again and again underscored, even emphasized
with italics within the decisions of the Supreme Court.
(Los Angeles vs Manhart, 1978)

Justice Marshall, certainly one who has been most sensitive to matters of this sort, has written in the strongest possible language that the provisions of the Civil Rights Act and of the equal protection clause apply to whites as well as blacks, and protect whites, and all other ethnic groups, as they protect blacks, in every way. (McDonald vs Santa Fe Trail Transportation Co., 1976)

No constitutional distinction can be drawn, therefore, which would retain the protections of the Fourteenth Amendment for some, but deny them for others. Honest or benign intentions to help one or another minority group cannot constitutionally justify discrimination on the basis of race. If the principle of the equal protection of the law applies, it applies to us all. Racial preference in professional school admissions is therefore a violation of our constitution.

4. Finally, racial preference in medical school admissions is wrong because it is injurious--hurtful to those displaced, of course, but hurtful also to the minorities it is supposed to assist, and hurtful to the entire society. (Regents vs Bakke, 1978; Cohen, 1979a)

Many who advocate racially preferential programs admit that they do not like them, find themselves queasy in their administration. But (say they) we've just got to do it because the results will be so awful if we don't. In fact, however, if we consider the results over the long run, racial preference is not good for anyone. Deliberate favoritism on grounds of race will plant--in fact, already has planted--the seeds of racial anger and racial tension for many years to come. It is of no benefit to our society to tamper with its fundamental principles of equal protection under the law. If we do tamper with this principle, we will reap the whirlwind.

Moreover, such programs will prove no lasting benefit to the minorities themselves, who are the object of the supposed assistance. It is no benefit to members of a minority group, blacks or Hispanics, to have their color or national origin attached, in the minds of all in society, to the notion of charity and payoff, and to the

suggestion of lesser competence. It is no benefit to the
reputations of superbly qualified minority professionals
to be thought by many, black and white, as having reached
their professional position only because they had been
given special favor.

Those who support programs of racial preference
often refer to them as medicine, bitter but necessary.
I submit that they are, in fact, poison--poison of a kind
similar to that which put our society in so painful a
condition. We are deeply unwise to administer more of
it to ourselves.

CHAPTER II: THE BAKKE DECISION

Racial preference in medical school admissions was
struck down in the famous case of The Regents of The
University of California vs Allan Bakke (1978). This
complicated and agonizing case, one that received more
public attention than any case in the history of the United
States Supreme Court, has unfortunately been very badly
reported. There is a great deal of confusion about what
the legal consequences are for the medical schools and for
those involved with admission to medical schools. The
confusion stems from an unusual configuration of Supreme
Court Justices in the actual rendering of the decision:
there were four Justices in one party, four Justices in
another, and a ninth Justice as a single party sharing
some of the positions of both. Four Justices held, as
I mentioned earlier, that the program at The University
of California at Davis (whose facts I do not need to
rehearse--sixteen seats in an entering class of 100 were
essentially set aside for minority groups) was simply
unlawful. They held that a minority program so devised,
reserving seats for members of minority groups exclusively,
however those minorities were defined, is a violation of
the Civil Rights Act. That (said they) closes the matter.
A fifth Justice, Justice Powell, argued that determining
whether or not such programs do violate the Civil Rights
Act required a constitutional analysis. Four other Justices
held that it was in fact not a violation either of the
Constitution or of the Civil Rights Act. Critical to the
whole decision, therefore, was the opinion of Justice

Powell, who announced the opinion of the Court, whose
opinion appears first, and whose opinion for all practical
purposes governs us in these matters. Justice Powell
held, in essence, that when one explores the meaning of
the equal protection clause in the Constitution of the
United States in order to find out what principles the
Civil Rights Act made concrete, one finds that all programs
which excluded on the basis of race are intolerable. Justice
Powell, with a certain amount of passion, but also with a
lengthy, careful review of the Davis program in all its
aspects, joins the four Justices who look only to the Civil
Rights Act in striking down that program as impermissible.
Bakke was ordered admitted to the University of California.

The results of the Bakke case have sometimes been
reported as follows: "Well, the Supreme Court struck
down rigid quotas, but it did not strike down affirmative action." This is a very misleading way in which
to describe the true state of affairs. If one means by
"affirmative action" the carefully tailored compensatory
relief for identifiably injured persons, it is certainly
true that the Court did not strike that down. If one
means by "affirmative action" (as many do who would like
to evade the impact of the Bakke decision) the continuation
of programs that give plain racial preference, that report
is simply a mistake. Racial preference in admissions--
not just rigid quotas, but all flat racial preference--
was forbidden by this decision.

It is true then, Justice Powell concluded in his
pivotal opinion, that it would be incorrect to say that
one could never under any circumstances attend to race in
determining admission to medical or professional schools.
That far he agreed with those Justices who supported the
Davis program, allowing that consideration of race might
under some circumstances be permissible. But, said Justice Powell, the circumstances under which race may be
permissibly considered are very few and very narrow. With
the Bakke decision before us we know, without speculation,
what the rules are now, and we have the obligation to
comply with the principles of Justice Powell's governing
opinion. He is, for the present, the gate-keeper for the

uses of race in college admissions; no admissions program
is permissible if it fails to heed the conditions he laid
down.

What conditions are these? They are specific pro-
hibitions respecting both the aims of any uses of race
in admission, and the means with which those aims are pursued.

One narrow purpose only, for Powell, justifies the use
of race in college admissions -- student diversity. Three
other goals often advanced to justify such programs he
explicitly rejected. (Regents v. Bakke, pp. 305-11)

(1) He firmly rejects a university's use of race "to
assure within its student body some specified percentage of
a particular group merely because of its race or ethnic
origin." That is plain racial discrimination, he explains,
and on its face is forbidden by the Constitution.

(2) A university might conceivably use race in admissions to improve professional services delivered to
communities presently underserved, but only if it could
prove that such use of race was necessary for that end; and
that, Powell concludes, has not been shown at all. Classification by race for preference in admission presently
appears to have no significant effect upon health care
delivery; until proved to have such an effect that justification of racial preference must also be rejected.

(3) Most importantly, universities may not consider
race in admissions for the purpose of helping certain groups
perceived as victims of societal discrimination. The end in
that case may be honorable but, Powell insists, it "does not
justify a classification that imposes disadvantages upon
persons like respondent [Bakke], who bear no responsibility
for whatever harm the beneficiaries of the special admissions program are thought to have suffered." A college has
no business, Powell tells us, giving advantages to members
of one race at the expense of disadvantaging members of
another race, to compensate for damages that the college
believes were done by society at large. Powell specifies
that racial preference, as a remedy for injustice, may be
given only where an institution has been found, by an
appropriate authority, to have violated the laws or the
Constitution to the harm of identifiable persons. Without

that finding, publicly supported institutions have no
adequate justification for inflicting the harm on those such
as Bakke that racially preferential admissions programs do.
Universities do not have the authority to grant, at their
pleasure, social remedies for some at the cost of injury to
blameless third parties. College admissions committees are
neither legislatures nor courts.

The one goal that may justify the use of race in admissions (but does not oblige that use) is "the attainment
of a diverse student body," (Regents v. Bakke, pp. 311-15)
a First Amendment interest fitting for a university in view
of its special functions. Colleges, Powell writes, have
"the right to select those students who will contribute the
most to 'the robust exhange of ideas,'" and they may consider ethnicity in admissions to advance that end -- but
only that end. It follows that attention to race is permissible only where a broad array of differing characteristics are, in fact, seriously and competitively weighed, "of
which racial or ethnic origin is just a single though important element." If the only diversity sought is among
ethnic groups, that will not by itself satisfy the First
Amendment value which alone may justify a consideration of
race normally forbidden. Powell is specific. A college
practice sensitive to the race of applicants must be concretely devised to achieve diversity on many dimensions.
Nor may administrators say that since diversity has long
been one of our objectives, business may go on as usual.
Powell is emphatic. We are permitted attention to race for
no reason other than diversity; and our service to diversity,
if race is involved, must be more than with our lips.

So much for the one goal that may justify the use of
race in admissions. The means to achieve that goal are also
narrowly restricted in the Powell opinion. Whatever system
a university employs, it must guarantee that what applies to
persons of one race applies equally to persons of every
other race. Powell is unequivocal on this point. "The
guarantee of equal protection cannot mean one thing when
applied to one individual and something else when applied to
a person of another color. If both are not accorded the
same protection, then it is not equal." Any program,
therefore, that utilizes a double standard openly or covertly,
or that excludes from the competition for any set of seats
or benefits any persons because of their ethnic features,
fails this constitutional test. It is not saved by the

good intentions of its authors. Any "system of allocating benefits and privileges on the basis of skin color and ethnic origin" manifests "inherent unfairness." Applicants for admission must be treated as individuals; any special program dealing with applicants by race exhibits a "fatal flaw."

The bearing of these principles on present practice is much greater than has been generally realized. Virtually all special admissions programs have been, in Powell's sense, fatally flawed. Most have maintained double lists and double standards, have categorized by color and ethnic origin to set screening levels and procedures. Many still do exclude whites, or white males, from competition for certain places or other benefits. Most special admissions programs were deliberately devised to deal with people by race. Their objectives, moreover, have commonly been the very ones Powell rejects as impermissible. Most were frankly designed to "assure...some specified percentage of a parti- cular group merely because of its race or ethnic origin." Whether by "goal" or by "quota" (a distinction Justice Powell dismisses as superficial) their targets have been racial or ethnic proportions---an aim Powell finds uncon- stitutional. Or they have been designed to compensate minorities for societal injury. Or they have been put forward as plans to compensate disadvantaged students, where "disadvantaged" commonly serves as a euphemism for black or brown in institutions embarrassed by plain racial discrim- ination. If Justice Powell's opinion is controlling, special admissions program may no longer be defended on those grounds. If those are the grounds on which they rest, explicitly or tacitly, such programs, at least in state-supported institu- tions, are not in compliance with the law of the land.

CHAPTER III: OBJECTIONS AND REPLIES

Objections to the Powell opinion are of two kinds. One concerns its merits: whether, after considering the many complexities of racially preferential admissions systems, he would have been wiser to adopt some other interpretation of the equal protection clause. Some would wish the governing interpretation more restrictive, precluding all uses of race. Some would wish it less restrictive, permitting more uses of race. But that issue (at least until it arises, if ever, in another admissions case) is now closed.

A second set of objections deal not with the substantive merit of the Powell opinion, but with its suitability as a set of governing principles for college admissions. Here the objections are of two sub-types, the first directed at the feasibility of the Powell principles, the second at their coherence. I deal with each of these issues in turn.

Feasibility is a proper concern, even for those who do not quarrel with the authority of the principles outlined above. Can professional schools, in view of the enormous number of applicants for very few places, seriously hope to treat each applicant as an individual and not as a member of a group? Is the demand that ethnicity be no more than one of many dimensions on which all applicants are evaluated singly a realistic one? If not, the Powell principles, however right in theory, will be abandoned in practice, not out of defiance but out of practical necessity.

One who has experienced the complexity and size of the admissions process at a fine college will appreciate the sincerity of this complaint. Principles that would govern a process must be applicable in practice. But this complaint is entirely answerable. In the first place, most colleges and universities are troubled now not by an excess of appli- cants, but by declining applications. Many institutions have faculties and residence halls larger than their present enrollments can justify. For a decade or more the decline is likely to continue. A number of private colleges are closing; some state colleges may follow suit. The problem of feasibility for the Powell principles seems greater than it is because of the general tendency to focus on a few premier colleges and professional schools where, indeed, applications outnumber places by twenty or thirty or more to one.

In these premier institutions, however, the Powell principles can be applied by conscientious admissions officers. Objectives other than diversity for the use of race must be eliminated; there is no difficulty in that. But how can ad- ministrators achieve diversity without bundling applications in groups: rural and urban, out-of-state and in-state, male and female, over 30 and under 30, black and brown and white, and so on? The identification of such characteristics will be entailed by a quest for diversity, but the process need not (and now it must not) center upon the division of ap- plicants into ethnic piles, and it must not be a process whose result is fashioned to reach certain numerical results with respect to those piles. Rather, the primary sorting will be by intellectual attainment or promise (or other characteristics reasonably linked to successful performance in the program in question) with subsidiary sortings by other characteristics that may reasonably be supposed to advance the aims of student diversity. Ethnicity may be one of these. The task is complicated. But the admissions process in such premier institutions must be complicated to be fair. There is nothing in the restrictions Powell lays down that cannot be readily incorporated in a just and rational admissions process.

Would that not impose a terrible burden of inconvenience and cost upon the college? No. Eliminating the double-standard system now commonly in use will effect substantial savings of time and energy. The treatment of ethnicity as but one of an array of subsidiary characteristics most of which are already considered will introduce no great addi-tional complexity, and can be fitted readily into most race-neutral systems.

But the ultimate answer to any complaint regarding the practical burden of Powell's principles is that, whatever the burden, it must be borne if ethnicity is to be weighed. The Supreme Court has laid down the ways in which race may be used in admissions if it is to be used at all. No college is obliged to consider race in admissions; a college may be well advised not to do so. But should it determine that diversity is essential, and that ethnic diversity is vital, the administrative costs in pursuing these goals lawfully may not serve to justify allegedly more convenient "two-class" systems that violate the equal protection guarantee of the Fourteenth Amendment.

A related objection touches upon the genesis of Powell's principles, and his alleged misapplication of them. The critic contends that Justice Powell mistakenly supposes that admissions criteria arising in a undergraduate context and applicable chiefly to schools of liberal arts must be applied equally to professional schools. Thus, he provides as a model for the consideration of race in a competitive medical school the admissions document from Harvard. Diversity may be an important consideration in undergraduate selection, but for the selection of future doctors or lawyers it has much reduced significance, perhaps none. To permit diversity

as the only ground for the use of race in such professional
contexts appears to exhibit a naive confusion.

Powell is neither naive nor confused on this point.
Any who register this criticism with condescension would do
well to study this portion of Powell's opinion more carefully.
(Regents v. Bakke,pp. 311-319) He is fully aware that the
need for diversity may vary with context. He believes (and
as former President of the American Bar Association he can
be said to have some understanding of the needs of the
professional schools) that diversity of students in the
class is a desideratum as important in medical and legal
education as in the liberal arts. Reasonable persons may
differ on this question. Powell's point, however, is that
if race is to be a factor in professional school admissions
it may be a factor for no other reasons. Where diversity is
believed a dimension of little import to medical or legal
education, admissions officers are at liberty to abandon it.
Powell, unlike some of his critics, is not searching for a
ground upon which the consideration of race is permissible.
Student diversity is that ground; ethnicity may enter the
admissions process in no other form.

That Powell's principles do not make sense, that they
cannot coherently achieve their aim, is a second sub-type of
complaint against them. Here also the thrust is practical,
the spirit sometimes derisive: everyone knows that under
the language of the Harvard admissions program (appended by
Powell to his opinion as an example of an admissions system
in which race enters only for the achievement of diversity)
a college can do precisely what the Davis Medical School did
through open racial preference. "The cynical," wrote Justice
Blackman in his dissenting opinion, "may say that under a
program such as Harvard's one may accomplish covertly what
Davis concedes it does openly." (Regents v. Bakke, p. 406)
Justice Brennan wrote similarly:

"That the Harvard approach does not also make
public the extent of the [racial] preference and the
precise workings of the system, while the Davis program
employs a specific, openly stated number, does not
condemn the latter plan....It may be that the Harvard
plan is more acceptable to the public than is the Davis
"quota."...But there is no basis for preferring a
particular preference program simply because in a
achieving the same goals that the Davis Medical

School is pursuing, it proceeds in a manner that is not immediately apparent to the public." (Regents v. Bakke, p. 379)

This objection to the Powell principles is profoundly mistaken. Certainly some may cheat. Surely some may, under the cover of a set of approved words, engage in a pattern of action whose hidden principles, if exposed, would be found impermissible. Some say that Harvard itself is guilty of such duplicity. But the example Powell has given is not what Harvard does, but what Harvard says it does, which is, precisely, to consider race for the attainment of student diversity, and for that purpose only. If in truth a school considers race in admissions for reasons other than diversity, it does wrong. We are all expected not to act so as to deceive the courts.

Between the Davis program and the Harvard program, Powell points out, there is this crucial difference: the former exhibits on its face an intent to discriminate by race, the latter does not. It is of course possible to adopt and present to the world language that reveals no discriminatory intent, and then, knowingly but covertly, to act with precisely the intention that is forbidden. The possibility of such subterfuge, although real, proves nothing. Frequent allusion to it suggests (unfairly, in my view) that admissions officers are a breed specially prone to employ unlawful chicanery to achieve their ends.

If one college uses the Harvard language honestly, and another college uses the same language to cheat, there is a sharp line of distinction between the conduct of the two. The boundary between them is the intent of their authors and administrators. One can picture Justice Powell deliberately looking at us and saying emphatically, as he writes near the conclusion of his long and thoughtful opinion: "And a Court would not assume that a university, professing to employ a non-discriminatory admissions policy, would operate it as a cover for the functional equivalent of a quota system. In short, good faith would be presumed." All university officers must hear themselves addressed by these words.

An objection to the Powell principles closely related to this one is presented by Ronald Dworkin. (Dworkin, 1978) Dworkin reasons as follows: to reserve certain places in

a medical school entering class for minorities only, while
opening the remainder to all, minority and majority, through
competition, is indeed to handicap the white, majority
applicant in some degree. But to weigh the blackness or
brownness of a minority applicant's skin as a plus factor in
a quest for diversity is also to handicap the white, majority
applicant to some degree. It cannot matter to the white
applicants which way they are handicapped. What is important to them is the degree of the handicap. It may prove
more to their advantage to be excluded from the competition
for a few seats reserved for minorities than to have a crack
at every seat yet be substantially handicapped by the
"diversity" factor. Justice Powell thus draws a distinction
without a real difference. He thinks that reserving places
for minority applicants is unfair, while giving "plus points"
for minority group membership is fair. But these are only
two ways of doing the same thing. It is the size of the
handicap imposed, the critic argues, not the mode of its
imposition, that really counts. Dworkin writes:

> "Whether an applicant competes for all or only
> part of the places, the privilege of calling
> attention to other qualifications does not in
> any degree lessen the burden of his handicap,
> if it is unfair at all. If the handicap does
> not violate his rights in a flexible plan [i.e.,
> one pursuing only diversity], a partial exclusion
> does not violate his rights under a quota. The
> handicap and the partial exclusion are only
> different means of enforcing the same fundament-
> al classifications. In principle, they affect
> a white applicant in the same way--by reducing
> his overall chances--and neither is, in any
> important sense, more "individualized" than the
> other. The point is not (as Powell once suggests
> it is) that faculty administering a flexible
> system may covertly transform it into a quota plan.
> The point is rather that there is no difference,
> from the standpoint of individual rights, between
> the two systems at all." (Dworkin, 1978 p. 23)

The complaint appears shrewd, but it rests upon a
fundamental misunderstanding of Powell's distinction between
the consideration of race as one factor in a quest for
diversity and plain racial preference. If our object were
simply to favor non-white applicants by imposing a "handicap"

on white applicants, there are many ways this could be accomplished. It can be accomplished by giving enough "plus points" for blackness or brownness to achieve the results desired. Any racial proportions antecedently chosen can be obtained by the manipulation of the diversity factor as well as by reserving places. But that use of diversity is fraudulent. To use diversity in that way is to do, under the cover of nondiscriminatory language, just what has been forbidden. Once we decide to handicap one racial group, the instrument is of no great consequence, save that some instruments are more detectable than others. But imposing a handicap on any ethnic group is precisely what is not permitted. Dworkin's reasoning reveals what his objective is: to save racial preference. But the intention to do that, either by reserving places or by manipulating the diversity factor, has been precluded by the Powell principles. Seeking diversity honestly is one thing; scheming under the name of diversity is another. Again, intent makes all the difference.

The critic may try to avoid this moral response by arguing that a handicap is simply a handicap; taken descriptively it involves no intent whatever. If minorities are advantaged in the quest for diversity because they are fewer, the majority is that far handicapped. That handicap (he may say) is intrinsically no different from one imposed deliberately by reserving places, irrespective of intent. If the degree of overall disadvantage is the same, intent makes no difference. The critic maintains that Powell is simply confused in believing that one system hurts the white majority unfairly while the other does not. Either both systems are unfair or neither is.

This version of the complaint is obtuse. An applicant is not treated unfairly when the characteristics he does or does not in fact possess are weighed, along with those of other applicants, in a system reasonably designed to choose the best entering class. If, in a medical school, diversity really is one consideration in the overall selection of the entering class, being in certain categories (having a rural background or indigent parents, being an experienced engineer or a Hawaiian, etc.) might reasonably be considered in one's favor, in small degree, after more fundamental intellectual characteristics had left some difficult choices before the admitting committee. When the unusual are favored, at the margins, the usual are disfavored that far. Everyone

understands that, and the good reasons for it. No one,
in that circumstance, is done injustice. When the members
of one race are favored, however, simply because of their
race, and the members of other races or ethnic groups disfavored by the same device, the matter is wholly different,
as our courts have made very plain. That is unjust and is
not to be tolerated.

In an honest quest for diversity one's race may be
considered in one's favor as an applicant. But so also
might one's family background be considered, or one's
artistic accomplishments, or economic circumstances, or any
other characteristics one possesses that may contribute to
the larger goals that diversity itself serves. Each applicant is just what he is: exhibiting just his own degree of
poise or poverty or whatever. There is all the difference
in the world between disadvantage arising out of ordinari-
ness, a marginal handicap every white male has the opportunity to overcome by exhibiting other features that enable
him to contribute richly to the class, and disfavor flatly
imposed because of one's race. Even if the degree of
disadvantage were to prove the same (a most improbable
outcome unless the diversity factor were being manipulated),
the ground of the disadvantage matters a very great deal:
racial preference is unfair in a way that advantage from
unusualness is not.

Nor may it be argued that, although honestly seeking
diversity, a scheme may be devised to consider only race
because the other elements of diversity (sex, age, geographical origins, etc.) are incorporated without special
attention. Diversity, this argument concludes, simply boils
down to racial diversity. This objection will not do
because, if diversity really is the honest aim of an individualized process, every applicant must have at least the
equal opportunity to strengthen the case for his admission
on the basis of diversity manifested in other ways. To
provide that opportunity a deliberate and conscious, not
incidental, attention must be paid to at least a substantial
range of applicant differences. The precise boundaries of
the range may vary, but without explicit attention to
manifold factors of which race is but one, diversity will
not have been employed in such a way as to meet the demand
of the Fourteenth Amendment that no person, viewed as an
individual, may be denied the equal protection of the laws.

Powell's principles are distinguished at bottom from attempted obfuscation or evasion by intent. He expects universities to act in good faith; this expectation cannot be emphasized too strongly. When explicit Supreme Court rules permit the use of race in admission for only certain purposes, and only in certain ways, institutions of higher learning have a powerful obligation to comply with the spirit of those rules. What we intend is part of the act governed by those principles.

In universities, of all places, intellectual integrity and civic responsibility must be sensitively and concretely honored. Devious schemes through which a college may satisfy the letter while evading the substance of its obligations are clearly not tolerable. Nor may a university respond to the law with procedures designed to obscure or mislead. Compliance must be unambiguous and forthright; for a university nothing less will be compliance in "good faith."

Universities that do not live up to this expectation will fail in their duty. They will also be acting most imprudently. College officers who hide impermissible ends with hypocritical language will surely answer for it. Admissions systems can no longer be shrouded in secrecy, as Bakke makes clear. Duplicity will not prove hard to expose. Institutions that connive to avoid the law will bring upon themselves the policing of their intra-institutional processes by government in ways more painful than any our universities have yet experienced, to the serious detriment of their larger purposes.

The belief that the Bakke decision, while striking down "rigid quotas," permits most university programs giving minority preferences without quotas to go on as usual is (as we have seen in reviewing Powell's principles) simply mistaken. State-supported racially preferentially admissions systems, whether incorporating quotas or goals, or using any other language, have been determined inadmissible. What was condemned by a majority of the Court in this case is not merely the instrument of quotas, but the system of favoritism by race of which it was the tool. Any tool having the same object is subject to the same comdemnation.

Is the Bakke decision, then, a serious blow to affirmative action in this sphere? That depends upon what one means by "affirmative action." If one means by it (as many now do) racial preference for minorities as such, the answer is yes. All of us, minorities most particularly, should give thanks for that. Institutionalized preference by race is not only unjust, but gravely damaging in the long run to those whom it purports to aid.

If by "affirmative action" we mean, however, what the phrase was originally intended to convey, the taking of positive steps to insure that earlier discriminatory practices were uprooted, the Bakke decision will advance, not deter, such action. To recruit from all sources fairly; to test fairly and without racial bias; to weigh merits (intellectual or other) on an individual basis, with all handicap flowing from race scrupulously eliminated--these affirmative steps the Bakke decision supports without dissent. It was not affirmative action in this wholesome, impartial sense that was at issue in this case. Favor by race was the issue; it was here condemned.

CHAPTER IV: CONCLUDING OBSERVATIONS

The long-term ramifications of the Bakke decision have been underestimated. Two themes embodied in it will reverberate for many years to come, contributing substantially to our constitutional history.

The first of these bears chiefly upon colleges and universities. They are forbidden by Bakke from using admissions standards to achieve societal objectives that are not properly in their sphere. Justice Powell writes:

> "We have never approved a classification that aids persons perceived as members of relatively victimized groups at the expense of other innocent individuals in the absence of judicial, legislative or administrative findings of constitutional or statutory violations.... Without such findings of constitutional or statutory violations it cannot be said that the government has any greater interest in helping one individual than in refraining from harming another.

> "Petitioner [the University of California] does not purport to have made, and is in no

position to make, such findings. Its broad
mission is education, not the formulation of
any legislative policy or the adjudication of
particular claims of illegality." (Regents v.
Bakke, pp. 307-309)

By this firm restriction we (I speak for the academic
world of which I am a member) are done a great service.
Universities have repeatedly and rightly argued that legislatures should not seek to use us, deform us, to achieve
political objectives foreign to our essential purposes. It
is incumbent upon us to restrain ourselves from that same
perversion. Restorative justice, taking from some and giving
to others to right social wrongs, is an enterprise universities and their admissions committees are not likely to be
very good at. But even if we are good at it, if our admissions officers were as well trained as judges, it is
still not our proper role. We are neither judges nor leg-
islators. It is simply wrong for us to exercise our powers
as though we were, conducting admissions policies not merely
as college functions but as a device to correct social
wrongs that we decide deserve remedy, at whatever costs to
other parties we deem reasonable.

If we announce that it is our business to set things
right in the world, what may we expect from legislatures
when we decline to serve as their political instrument in
some other context they deem pressing? Shall we tell them
then that ours is an educative mission, and that we ought
not be made tools of social policy? Can we then expect to
be taken seriously? Once the principle is accepted--indeed
is urged by us--that we, the universities, are a proper
court in equity, to take from X and give to Y to remedy his-
torical social wrongs, we will face a host of moral and
political claims, many entirely reasonable, upon which we
shall have the same obligation to act. What a dreadful
disservice that will be, both to education and to justice.
Justice Powell, in forbidding this course to us, saves us
from our over-zealous selves. He takes the non-political
nature of higher education seriously, as we, in our sober
moments, also do. His protection of the universities from
self-assignment into political or juridical service is
likely to prove, in the years ahead, a feature of the Bakke
decision for which all will be grateful.

The second positive theme of Bakke, very much neglected,

concerns societal attention to race. The case is not the landmark sought by either side, though it should not be forgotten that Bakke won. Yet there is an important message in the decision to American society, one critical theme, much overlooked, upon which the entire Supreme Court is there in agreement. It is this: persons like Allan Bakke, when displaced or disadvantaged by a racially preferential system, are injured. They are done constitutional injury in being deprived of what they ordinarily would not have been deprived of under the Constitution.

All nine Supreme Court Justices are in accord on this, not just the four Justices of the Stevens group, not just they and Powell. The Brennan group, although approving the Davis plan, agrees throughout that Bakke was substantially hurt, and that his hurt was serious enough to require very solid justification. Justice Blackman, one of the anti-Bakke four, writes in his separate opinion that he looks forward to the time when "persons will be regarded as persons, and discrimination of the type we address today [i.e., against Bakke] will be an ugly feature of history... that is behind us." (Regents v. Bakke, p. 403)

Reverse discrimination, in sum, is real and bad. In Bakke, for the first time, the Supreme Court had recognized that reality explicitly, and has made very clear to all that such discrimination, however well-intended, is not to be taken lightly. Until Bakke there were many who assumed that, so long as intentions were good, universities could act pretty much as they thought just, giving and taking as they pleased. Not so. There are those, including some on the Supreme Court, who believe that some reverse discrimination can be justified. But the lasting impact of the Bakke decision, practical and symbolic, is this: the advocates of racial discrimination face a mighty burden of proof. When, as in most contexts, that burden cannot be met in court, colleges and universities are well advised to avoid scrupulously all preference by race.

Finally, there is one troubling aspect of the Bakke decision that flows directly from the Powell principles. Not the restrictiveness of the result, but the invitation it may be taken to proffer, could lead to unhappy practices. In Bakke we are told that the Constitution permits the consideration of race in admissions for the sake of diversity, to further the First Amendment interest in free expression.

That being so, it would appear that other classifications as suspect as race--political affiliation or religion--may also be used for the sake of diversity. This is a disquieting result. Should the fact that one is a Republican or a Socialist, Catholic or Jew, be allowed to count in the distribution of opportunities? Surely we will answer that, even if counting such considerations did increase diversity in some contexts, they ought never be factors in the apportionment of any public goods. History gives us powerful grounds to conclude that the use of such classifications, even for putatively honorable goals, is an invitation to disaster. We forswear it. Then, even if Bakke permits it to achieve diversity in a student body, perhaps it will be the part of wisdom to foreswear the use of race as well.

REFERENCES

City of Los Angeles v Manhart 435 US702, at 708 (1978).
Cohen C (1980). Equality, diversity, and good faith. Wayne Law Rev 26(4):1261.
Cohen C (1975). Honorable ends, unsavory means. The Civil Liberties Review 2(2):106.
Cohen C (1979a). Justice debased: The Weber decision. Commentary 68(3):43.
Cohen C (1977). Race and equal protection of the laws. Lincoln Law Rev 10(2):117.
Cohen C (1980). What is "affirmative action?" Tex Law Rev 58:845.
Cohen C (1979b). Why racial preference is illegal and immoral. Commentary 67(6):40.
Dworkin R (1978). The Bakke decision: Did it decide anything? New York Review of Books Aug. 17,p. 23.
McDonald v Santa Fe Trail Transportation Co. 427 US 273, (1976) pp. 278-83.
Regents of the University of California v Allan Bakke, 438 US 256 (1978).
Title VI, Civil Rights Act of 1964; Sec 601, 42 USC#2000d (1970).

**Troubling Problems in Medical Ethics: The Third
Volume in a Series on Ethics, Humanism, and Medicine: 39–45**
© **1981 Alan R. Liss, Inc., 150 Fifth Ave., New York, NY 10011**

AFFIRMATIVE ACTION IN MEDICAL SCHOOL ADMISSIONS

H. Jack Geiger, M.D.
Arthur C. Logan Professor of Community Medicine
Sophie Davis School of Biomedical Education
The City College of the City University of NY
New York, New York

Let me begin with a reiteration of a point that was
made by the first speaker. This is not an argument. This
is not an adversary situation. We start with the presumption
that we are all interested in equity and justice, and we
recognize that there are many ways to look at this problem.
I am reminded of this because I am going to talk about some
things that have already been addressed, but a great many
that haven't been, and from quite a different perspective.
Professor Cohen began looking at the specific cases that
were presented to us for our consideration, and turned almost
at once to say, "Let's see if we can identify the issues
that are implicit in these cases, the issues that underlie
this whole area." My approach to the identification of this
set of issues is, however, different from that which rests
on the body of law and political tradition (all of which I
quite agree is relevant). I think we have a set of unanswered
questions, and that these cases quite clearly indicate that
they are unanswered questions. Let me identify some of them.

First: is admission to medical school a private or
merit good, or a public or social good? That is, is
admission a reward, earned on the basis of individual merit
and to be handed out as a good to those competing for it,
or is it a good to be distributed in accordance with some
plan for fulfilling social purposes and social needs? Or
is it an uneasy, ill-defined mix of both? Or is it in the
actual process of medical school admissions, a stacked deck?
Our answer to this question--private or public, merit or
social--has a great deal to do with our definitions of what
is equitable and fair.

Furthermore, how shall this good be distributed in a society that is in other ways demonstrably inequitable in terms of the distribution of its opportunities, goods, and resources?

Next we must ask whether the criteria of merit are relevant. Are they equitable? The criteria of merit are terribly important factors in decisions as to how resources shall be distributed. What is the social context in which we are making these decisions? Are medical schools and universities unique institutions, or should they be regulated as a part of the overall social process? What social context should we strive for in terms of the distribution of opportunities, of health and illness, of medical care, and of resources? How do we balance attempts to reduce inequities in the societal distribution of health or illness (or at least of medical care resources) against concepts of individual rights, or the different conceptions of fairness at the point of entry to medical school?

I am going to address broad issues, but let me refer you to "DOUBLE INDEMNITY: The Poverty and Mythology of Affirmative Action in the Health Professional Schools," by Hal Strelnick, M.D., and Richard Younge, M.D. of the Health Policy Advisory Committee, (1980) which has, I think, the best overall summary of some of the factual data concerning admissions. Much of the data I will present comes from this publication.

Since 1974, minority admissions and minority representation in medical school and other health professional schools has been stable or actually declining, contrary to a public impression. But there is an issue in addition to ethnicity or race, and that is social class. To be lower social class is very often to be educationally disadvantaged. Social class is highly correlated with race and ethnicity, although not coterminous with it. We are in part talking about a maldistribution of positions by social class, which has racial and ethnic consequences.

According to the most recent data I've seen, 48% of the places in medical school classes in the United States are now occupied by students from families in the top 4% of the population with respect to income. When one looks at the other end of the spectrum, the situation is exactly reversed; the very substantial number of people at the bottom of the income ladder have a very limited number of the places in medical school. It is this distribution, probably more than issues of race or ethnicity per se, that is skewing the selection process.

I would argue that our admission process as it exists now, particularly in terms of its definition of merit, represents a stacked deck. First of all, people from lower social class segments of the population, from the bottom of the economic social ladder, generally never get the kinds of educational opportunity that even lead them to the application process for medical school. In addition to their economic difficulties, most such students attend inferior schools in which the per capita public educational expenditure per student is significantly less than in other schools. By and large, you have to be upper middle class to make it to medical school. What are the experiences that facilitate acceptance? To be upper middle class; to go to a school with a high per capita budget, in a middle class community; to go to a high school which is geared toward producing college entrants; to go to a college rich in faculty, facilities and other resources (and not, for example, to a long-segregated Southern black college); to go to a college which trains students specifically to make their way through the pre-med jungle. All these are in the main prerogatives of the upper middle class which are denied to less wealthy aspirants to medical school. There is, in effect, a process beginning in Kinder-garten that stacks the deck long before we are faced with the set of eight choices and two places in our discussion case. One can argue that we need to treat people equally in the admissions process, that academic "merit" is the only criterion, and that we do damage by setting up preference systems. But to make the fundamental argument that everyone should be treated equally by an admissions committee is rather like saying: "In the name of equity, fairness and justice, we will have this 1000-yard race, but for the preceding month, 40% of the contestants will be allowed only 500 calories a week, with no protein, while the other 60% may have all the steak they want. However, from the starting line on, everyone will be treated equally."

Furthermore, even leaving aside the issue of unequal antecedent opportunity, I have considerable question about the definitions of merit. I would argue that these too constitute a stacked deck, biased by social class and other concerns. I would argue further that there is astonishingly little evidence of their relevance to social purpose.

Having served on medical school admissions committees for 15 years now, I think it is a fair statement (not as true as it used to be, but still fair) that an admissions committee consists of a group of medical school faculty members who are trying, with the best will in the world, to clone themselves. Their definitions of quality, by and large, use themselves, their peers and their colleagues as models. They rely heavily not only on things like MCAT scores and grade point averages but also on a considerable variety of social class cues. Again, I think social class turns out to be more important than race or ethnicity per se, but they overlap. These same committees may indeed be eager to admit minority students if they are middle class or upper middle class with good "merit" qualifications but these criteria, which usually go unquestioned, have relatively little demonstrated relevance to the important social purposes at the end. MCAT scores, for example, have a correlation with success in medical school, but most of that correlation is with success in the first two (basic science) years of medical school. In four of the five studies that I have been able to find which have compared quality of performance in practice to class standing in medical school, MCAT scores and all the rest, these correlations are almost nonexistent.

Common sense, if nothing else, tells us that there is obviously a minimum standard of competence required for medical education, a minimum level of knowledge and ability that should bar access to admission. But there is almost no evidence that the difference between being at that level and being at the high end of the spectrum correlates well with quality or performance in practice. Yet these criteria (MCAT scores, grade point averages and the like) are not only used as definitions of merit, but are also defended as predicting the "quality" of the students selected.

I have some personal experience of this, if I may be anecdotal. When I was at Tufts and working in Mississippi, we made an arrangement which indeed violates many of the principles defended earlier by Professor Cohen. We set up a separate admissions committee and said in effect that it would admit seven students a year from black rural Mississippi. We accepted seven students in each of two years. They were students who would never even have been interviewed, had they been judged by the usual criteria. Almost all were from southern black colleges. Almost all had MCAT scores under 300 (under the old system, when one generally needed about

575 even to get an interview, let alone be admitted). Yet
all had average or good grades in these relatively poor
colleges, and we felt they all had the capacity to make it.
These fourteen students were admitted under separate programs,
which indeed had the effect of denying places to a variety
of people "better qualified" according to conventional standards of merit, people who in turn had had prior advantages
in terms of educational opportunity.

During the first two years, the basic science years,
those fourteen students were clustered at the bottom of the
class; several had to repeat a year. The correlation between
their MCAT scores and their basic science performance was
indeed as predicted. Then we looked at their performance
during the clinical years. Almost without exception, they
were clustered at the junction of the bottom third and the
middle third of the class. It took me a while to realize
that this meant that they were performing better in the
clinical years than one third of the students admitted by
conventional criteria. Furthermore, it turns out that 13
of the 14 are back in Mississippi; one of them, in fact, is
my successor as director of the health center there at which
I worked for many years.

This raises a very difficult issue that is also implicit
in our cases this morning. Many admission officers are
concerned about applicants' plans for their medical careers
and their commitments to community and society.

There seems to be an implicit presumption that admission
of minorities to medical school is going to produce physicians
who will take care of minorities. By and large this has a
factual basis: most of the minority physicians in the United
States are mainly taking care of minority populations.
Minority populations are disproportionately served by the
available minority physicians. But there is an important
ethical question here. We seem to be saying, "Hey, minority
student, if we admit you, if you get through the chicken
wire, then you (unlike your colleagues) are particularly
obligated to serve minority communities, to be in the inner
city, to be in a set of situations which we know on other
grounds represent more limited financial opportunities and
represent more limited educational, academic, and professional
opportunities. Minority health is not a general social
responsibility, it is your specific responsibility because
your are a minority."

People who have been on my side, if there is a side (it's not that simple) of this issue, have in effect been working both sides of the street. Part of our argument has been that a powerful reason for the admission of more minority students to professional training is the possibility of the ultimate correction of inequities in the distribution of health care in the population. Yet, at the same time, we are usually the same people who say that the health of disadvantaged populations is a general social responsibility.

Social context is important in this. I think our consideration of admissions processess might be different if we had a national health service or if there were a general social obligation, for a significant part of every physician's career, as to where he or she would work.

But even this would not resolve completely these issues of general and antecedent social inequity in admission to medical school, or the biases in our definitions of merit, or the biases that operate on the basis of social class. I think we must find other ways to choose medical students. We could have not merely affirmative action, but--indeed--quotas.

We could set a floor, in terms of academic qualification, MCAT score, grade point average, educational preparation, and the like, and say, "yes, the evidence is very clear that without reaching this or that level of competence, people are not going to succeed in medical education and have a poor probability of becoming good physicians; but above that floor, let us have a lottery." The Dutch have been doing that for 10 years. Admission to medical school in Holland is by lottery from among all those above a minimum level of qualification. Yet as far as I can determine the quality of Dutch medical education and the quality of Dutch medical performance is equal to our own.

We could have a stratified lottery, with places reserved for the disadvantaged. There are still other alternatives or mixes of those plans that could be available to us.

This leads us at last to the purpose of medical schools. What is and is not the business of medical schools? Are they merely intellectual institutions pursuing their intellectual and academic business? Are there risks in involving them in social processess and asking them to fulfill social purposes in what might be called compensatory relief?

I argue that medical schools are now <u>perpetuating</u> the personal and social injustices for which we must seek compensatory relief. Medical schools exist for purposes beyond the intellectual and academic. Their other major functions are social. They exist to improve health care and its delivery. They obviously cannot do everything in this regard, but they have a major role to play in the construction of a health care system. Medical schools exist to meet a major social need, and ivory tower arguments simply won't work, and shouldn't work. If medical schools exist to meet that need, then it seems to me they need to be participants in more effective ways to reduce inequities: inequities of opportunity, of social class, of disadvantage, which means also, in our society, of race and ethnicity.

REFERENCES

(1) Strelnick H, Younge R (1980). "Double Indeminity: The Poverty and Mythology of Affirmative Action in the Health Professional Schools." New York: Health Policy Advisory Committee Special Report.

**Troubling Problems in Medical Ethics: The Third
Volume in a Series on Ethics, Humanism, and Medicine: 47–48
© 1981 Alan R. Liss, Inc., 150 Fifth Ave., New York, NY 10011**

DISCUSSION SUMMARY: AFFIRMATIVE ACTION IN MEDICAL SCHOOL
                       ADMISSIONS

Doreen L. Ganos
Director for Publicity and Registration, CEHM
University of Michigan
Ann Arbor, Michigan

All the participants rejected the use of a quota in deciding medical school admissions, considering it unfair and demoralizing. As one student stated, "Every human being deserves the dignity of being considered as an individual and not just a faceless type." A random lottery for all applicants fulfilling some basic academic standards was also rejected by almost all (98%) of the discussants, indicating their agreement that there are other criteria which must be applied to the admissions process.

The problem of identifying and ranking those criteria was far more controversial, however. In general, the groups divided possible criteria into two groups, those relating to individual merit, and those pertaining to societal benefit. Considering merit, all the groups agreed that some minimal level of MCAT scores and GPA was necessary. The discussants argued, however, as to how low such a standard ought to be in the face of such extenuating circumstances as a disadvantaged socioeconomic background. For example, some rejected Celia Jones (GPA 2.9) because "the minimum qualification should be at a 3.0" while others wanted to accept her over applicants with higher scores because she "worked hard against the odds." Although one group insisted that academic achievements should be the only basis for merit judgments, the rest asserted that other personal qualities should be included because they were "important indicators of how good a physician one would be." Some of the characteristics advanced as relevant were maturity, sensitivity to others, prior exposure to medicine, and strength of motivation.

Concerning the applicability of considerations of societal benefits to the medical school admissions process, all the groups decided that medical school training is a public as well as private good. They were quite concerned with the need for physicians in underserved areas and the amount of government support given to medical education. While 25% of the participants rated this consideration secondary to the merit criteria, the other 75% suggested that the fulfillment of social goals was at least of equal importance as the applicant's merit, so long as some minimal standard of merit was satisfied. Information considered relevant included where the applicant intended to practice, what specialty he thought he might choose, and what sort of a "social conscience" he seemed to have.

The groups also considered how the applicant's race and socioeconomic status should affect the admission process. All argued that low socioeconomic status can occasionally be considered as an extenuating circumstance in merit-oriented decisions, and that aiding the social advancement of such disadvantaged applicants is a desired social good. Interestingly, the groups were just as unanimous in rejecting race as a consideration, stating that race per se is not a relevant quality, and that as a measure of socioeconomic status (which is relevant) it is too imprecise. Discussants believed that socioeconomic disadvantages must be determined directly when these are used as an admissions criterion.

In concluding the discussion, each group applied their criteria to the case at hand, choosing two of the eight applicants. Half the groups voted to admit Celia Jones, and one third admitted Alex Miller. Sherwin Williams, Leon Johnson, and Sharon Goldman were all admitted by one sixth of the groups, with the last two the close third choice of another sixth. Bill Tane was not admitted by any, though he was the third choice of one sixth. Lastly, Bobby Chi and James Martin were not strongly considered for admittance by any of the groups.

**Troubling Problems in Medical Ethics: The Third
Volume in a Series on Ethics, Humanism, and Medicine: 49–51
© 1981 Alan R. Liss, Inc., 150 Fifth Ave., New York, NY 10011**

INTRODUCTION: DRUG TESTING IN PRISONS

Laurie Winkelman
Assistant Program Director, CEHM
University of Michigan
Ann Arbor, Michigan

Traditional theories of ethics are divided over the
issue of drug testing in prisons. The often quoted first rule
of medicine, "First do no harm," would tend to side against
such testing. Kantian theory, which says that each person
must be treated as an end rather than a means, also opposes
research which treats people as objects for study. In
contrast, a utilitarian would support experimentation in
prisons because such testing yields extensive benefits with
minimal risks. A libertarian might contend that every
person, prisoner or not, has the right to decide for himself
whether he would like to participate in drug testing.

Marx Wartofsky believes that drug experimentation in
prisons creates a moral dilemma. This dilemma stems from
our desire to produce medical and social benefits while
respecting human rights. Wartofsky believes that human
rights are violated when prisoners are coerced into participating in drug testing. He asserts, furthermore, that
coercion is indeed present in the current prison testing
scheme. He points particularly to the provision of less
stressful and higher quality living conditions for participating prisoners, to the significant monetary inducements
offered, and to the mistaken notion often held by prisoners
that participation improves chances for parole or reduction
of sentence. Wartofsky believes that drug testing in prisons
is unjust because the percentage of prisoners who participate
is much higher than the percentage of nonprisoners who do so
in experiments outside the prison system. He also objects
because most of the prisoners who do take part in these
studies are black and/or poor.

Wartofsky then describes four possible ways to resolve this dilemma. First, we can modify our idealistic approach to human rights so that it permits some prison experimentation. Second, we could preserve our idealism, but recognize its demands as guides to improvement rather than as absolute necessity. Third, we can continue with the current system of prison experimentation because the benefits to society justify violations of human rights. Fourth, we could discontinue all prison drug testing, even if this results in less accurate testing of new drugs, because we believe our respect for human rights to take precedence.

Wartofsky recognizes that drug testing in prisons is not going to be eliminated. Instead, he recommends the second approach, that we do the best we can to improve the system toward the ideal. He suggests prisoner representation on research planning and review committees to help assure that prisoners have the opportunity for voluntary and informed consent.

Robert Levine served as special consultant to the National Commission for the Protection of Human Subjects of Biomedical and Behavioral Research, which supported research that has the "...intent and reasonable probability of improving the health or well being of the individual prisoner." (Branson, 1977). As Levine explains, participation by prisoners in drug experimentation entails only an impressively small risk of complications. In fact, Levine believes that there is more danger involved in being a hospital patient than in being a therapeutic research subject.

Levine explains that pharmaceutical companies are not intentionally exploiting prisoners, for the monetary compensation that the prisoners receive is appropriate within the context of the prison economy. Levine believes that salaries for all of the jobs in the prison economy are economically exploitive. To improve the situation for the prisoners who are research subjects, he suggests that the pharmaceutical companies might place money in a general fund for the prisoners' welfare in addition to paying individual prisoners. Alternatively, prisoner subjects might be paid commensurately with non-prisoner subjects, but in order to avoid coercion, most of the money could be kept in an escrow account until the prisoners are released.

Pat Duffy, an inmate of Jackson Prison, elucidates the

differences between life inside and outside of prison. He
remarks that prisoners experience loss of individuality and
that life in prison is a constant struggle for survival,
covered by a facade of toughness. Duffy regards drug experimentation as a positive aspect of prison existence. Time
spent on the studies is time spent outside the hazardous
prison yard, and thus helps the prisoner retain his sanity.
Those participating in the studies benefit from complete
physicals and the highest wages in the prison. Duffy feels
sufficient information is given to the convicts about the
studies and that coercion is not a factor. He also denies
that the convicts would hide drug-related complications for
fear of being eliminated from the experiment. Duffy presents
a unique viewpoint and complements the analyses of the other
two speakers. However, it must be recognized that Duffy
himself was handpicked by the Jackson prison authorities and
experimenters for this presentation.

Our case for this topic focuses upon whether pharmaceutical companies should be allowed to conduct Phase I drug
testing in prisons. If this right is granted, we must also
ask what level of drug-associated risk is acceptable.
Research in prisons is currently restricted by the Department
of Health and Human Services to that from which individual
prisoners will likely obtain health benefits or to that
which studies the factors of prison life.

REFERENCES

Branson R (1977). Prison research: National Commission
    says, "No, unless. . ." Hasting Center Report 7(1):15.

Troubling Problems in Medical Ethics: The Third
Volume in a Series on Ethics, Humanism, and Medicine: 53-55
© 1981 Alan R. Liss, Inc., 150 Fifth Ave., New York, NY 10011

DRUG TESTING IN PRISONS

CASE FOR DISCUSSION

Phase I drug testing represents the first time a drug
is tested on humans. It aims at ascertaining only safety
and side effects and therefore is generally performed using
healthy volunteers. Prisons are attractive sites for Phase
I drug testing for two reasons. First, the population under
study can be easily controlled as necessary. They are
isolated in special living areas and thus protected from
many complicating variables. Second, volunteers are plentiful
and cheap in the prison setting, as there is little else to
do and prison medical compounds are often the best living
accommodations available to prisoners. While one hundred
dollars per day might be given to a non-prison volunteer for
such work who is confined to a hospital for continuous
monitoring, prisoners receive minimal compensation. Typical
fees include 50 cents to one dollar per day plus two dollars
for a complete physicial examination, one dollar per blood
sample, and 25 cents to three dollars per dose of a drug.

You are the director of the Detroit State Prison, a
newly built facility intended to reduce overcrowding at the
Jackson penitentiary. Jackson is one of the few prisons in
the country in which Phase I drug testing is being done and
the researchers at Upjohn and Parke Davis are quite eager to
add Detroit Prison to this list.

Dr. Donald O'Connor, the Director of Research at Upjohn,
proposes to study a longacting and highly potent analog of
phenytoin (an anti-epileptic drug). The Depo-phenytoin would
probably not offer intrinsically better seizure control than
phenytoin itself in the compliant patient, but it could be

useful in the treatment of poorly compliant patients who
would come in for a monthly injection rather than taking
pills three times per day. Animal testing has been unremark-
able except for apparently transient and reversible liver
toxicity in two monkeys out of five hundred tested. The
reported side effects of phenytoin itself in humans include
skin rashes, softening of bones, worsening of tendencies to
diabetes, nausea, vomiting, constipation, confusion and
slurring of speech, dizziness, increased hair growth, swelling
of the gums, and, rarely, cardiac arrhythmias occasionally
even resulting in death.

Parke Davis has an exciting new chemotherapeutic agent
which might be effective against bronchogenic (lung) and
certain other cancers. Animal studies have been promising
with good survival rates in unresectable tumors, but three
baboons out of two hundred tested developed serious impair-
ment of their immune systems. Two recovered and one died
from uncontrolled infection. The physician who did the
study notes that had the baboon been human, his life could
probably have been saved with advanced techniques too expensive for use on a baboon.

In each case, prisoners volunteering for the study
would be confined to a special wing of the prison hospital
(built with donations by the pharmaceutical companies).
They would receive three meals a day of infirmary food
(better tasting and more nutritious than ordinary prison
fare) and would in addition be offered the daily remuneration
of $4 for the chemotherapy study and one dollar for the
depo-phenytoin study (sizable sums in the prison economy).
They would be warned that participation or refusal to participate would not influence the quality of medical care they
receive in prison or their treatment by prison officials.
Volunteering would not be counted in favor of parole. They
would be told that they were free to quit the study at any
time without prejudice. All dangers and possible side effects
of the medication to be tested would be explained. All this
would be documented in a written informed consent. Each
prisoner would receive a complete medical workup in advance
and those at special risk would be eliminated from the
study. Prisoners would receive either drug or placebo for a
21 day period at appropriate dosages and neither prisoner
nor doctor would know who was getting which agent.

Trying to evaluate the possible risks of such studies,

you come upon a paper describing the complications of the
Jackson program (where anticancer drugs and other potentially
highly toxic agents are specifically excluded). (Zaraphonetis,
et al., 1978.) Common problems included allergic reactions,
dizziness, headache, nausea, and skin rashes. More serious
side effects were rare although one prisoner developed a
permanently deformed hip, one had a seizure and other significant toxicity occurred occasionally. All in all, out of
29,162 participants, 64 developed "significant medical
events." Another study (on non-prisoner subjects) reported
a 0.1% risk of "temporarily disabling" complications, one
patient with "permanently disabling complications", and no
fatalities in 93,399 subjects of non-therapeutic experimentation (Cardon, et al., 1976). You learn that the average
length of participation in a non-therapeutic study is three
days among non-prisoners and 21 days among prisoners.

Your associates and superiors in the Department of
Corrections have indicated formally that they will abide by
whatever you decide in this matter. The prisoners, many
former Jackson inmates, are either enthusiastic or at least
do not object to the program being available for others.
Will you recommend a policy permitting Phase I drug testing
in your prison? If so, would you approve either or both of
the proposed studies? Are there any additional restraints
or additional safeguards you would like to add? If not,
would you permit other drug testing? Therapeutic research?
Why (if at all) is experimentation different in the prison
setting and how does this affect your decisions?

(Case prepared by Laurie Winkelman and Marc D. Basson.)

Troubling Problems in Medical Ethics: The Third
Volume in a Series on Ethics, Humanism, and Medicine: 57–72
© **1981 Alan R. Liss, Inc., 150 Fifth Ave., New York, NY 10011**

THE PRISONERS' DILEMMA: DRUG TESTING IN PRISONS AND THE
VIOLATION OF HUMAN RIGHTS

Marx Wartofsky
Boston University
Boston, Massachusetts

1. INTRODUCTION: THE PRISONERS' DILEMMA

Under present conditions, the use of prisoners in non-
therapeutic pharmaceutical testing poses a moral dilemma. I
am going to try to present this dilemma in its sharpest
terms and then explore whatever alternative ways there may
be of escaping it or resolving it. I will argue that under
the present forms of such testing, it is inescapable and un-
resolvable, and that a resolution therefore lies either in
giving up such testing in prisons altogether or in changing
the conditions under which it takes place.

In its simplest form, the dilemma is this: either
testing proceeds as it is presently organized, and the
medical and social benefits of such testing are purchased at
the cost of violating the human rights of prisoners who are
the subjects of such testing, and specifically violating the
requirement of free and informed consent in experimentation
with human subjects; or the human rights of the prisoners
are observed at the cost of giving up the medical and social
benefits which result from such testing. We may restate the
dilemma somewhat more formally as follows: from the general
premise

(a) that one ought to do what is morally desirable and
refrain from doing what is morally undesirable,

and the subsidiary premises

(b) that it is morally desirable to observe human rights
and morally undesirable to violate them,

(c)   that it is morally desirable to produce medical and social benefits, and morally undesirable to fail to produce them where it is possible to do so,

(d)   1. that present forms of drug testing in prisons both violate the human rights of prisoners and specifically the requirements for free and informed consent, and
2. that present forms of drug testing in prisons also produce medical and social benefits,

the dilemma may be seen as follows: if we do what is morally desirable, then, at the same time, we do what is morally undesirable; and if we refrain from doing what is morally undesirable, then we also fail to do what is morally desirable. We are, in the classic dilemmatic terms, damned if we do and damned if we don't.

The burden of the dilemma may be seen to fall on only one of the premises, namely on premise (d), for premises (a), (b), and (c) seem unexceptionable. Therefore, any argument that this is, in fact, a dilemma, or any argument for escaping or resolving the dilemma will depend on an examination of both parts of premise (d): namely, (1) is it the case that drug testing in prisons violates the human rights of prisoners? and (2) does such drug testing in fact produce medical and social benefits? The major part of what follows in this paper will be concerned with these questions. But before proceeding, I want to generate the dilemma in still other terms, in order to characterize it further; and also to say some things about dilemmas in general.

We may see this dilemma as a counterposition of two approaches: the first I will call an ideal or normative approach, and the second, a realistic or meliorative approach to the use of prisoners in drug testing. The ideal approach concerns the moral imperative to observe human rights, without consideration of costs, or countervailing benefits which would accrue from violating these rights. The realistic or meliorative approach concerns the moral imperative to do whatever will, on the whole, improve human life, taking into account the ratio of benefit to cost, and therefore ordering relative values of what will produce greatest benefit at least cost. In the case at hand, the medical benefits of prison testing, and the social benefits of such programs to the prisoners would count in the balance against some degree of risk involved in the testing of new drugs. The question

is, however, would such benefits count, in the balance,
against violations of rights? On the other hand, can a right
be so sacrosanct that the improvement of health or of human
life should be sacrificed for it?

Here, we may be said to be involved in a practical
dilemma between an ideal norm and a realistic prospect of a
social good or of what is practically feasible. In practical
terms, does such an ideal norm become impossible to achieve,
or does its achievement require such stringent conditions that
it is practically unreasonable? Are we in the situation where
what we believe to be morally required is practically un-
feasible or impossible? The situation I am describing does
exist for a wide range of moral principles which we recognize
as attainable in practice only to some degree and never perfectly. That is, we hold to such principles as regulative
ideals, but we recognize that in our imperfections and within
the limits of practical life, they can only be approximated
and not fully realized. Perfect justice, the sanctity of
life, honesty, moral integrity, truthfulness, consideration
of others, equality in all our dealings with others -- these
begin the list of such ideals which are never perfectly realized. Is there a dilemma, then, between the commitment to
such ideals (which is widely shared), and the practical impossibility of realizing them? If there is such a dilemma
here, then it lies in the distinction between a normative or
ideal principle or a moral imperative, on the one hand, and
on the other, the impossibility of attaining it for practical
reasons, or because of practical imperatives which are overriding.

This is a different case from the dilemma in which there
is a conflict between two equally desirable, or equally requisite moral values, or between two moral imperatives; for
instance, between telling the truth or saving a life, or between being just and being merciful, or sacrificing one life
to save another. Here, the dilemma is either rationally un-
resolvable (if in fact there are only two mutually exclusive
options, each of which is equally weighty in its moral claims);
or it is "resolved" by random choice or the flip of a coin,
since the alternatives are indifferent. It cannot be resolved
by an ordering of these values, as to which overrides the
other, since, by hypothesis, they are equal.

This sort of dilemma can be formulated as a conceptual
or logical dilemma, since it does not concern differences in

what is practically feasible, but only a choice between two
equally imperative and equally feasible, though mutually exclusive, alternatives. The classical logical dilemmas are of
this sort. Thus, the traditional case of Buridan's Donkey
exemplifies this sort of dilemma (though it is not a moral
dilemma, but one concerning rational choice): The donkey is
equidistant from two identical bales of hay. Thus, there is
no more reason to choose to go to one rather than the other.
Stymied by this equivalence of rational options, the poor donkey has no grounds to choose one bale rather than the other,
and starves to death. Now we may answer that in a situation of
such perfect indifference, tossing a coin or choosing randomly
is the rational as well as the practical option, while starving
to death is not. There is no practical dilemma here, at any
rate, since each bale of hay is equivalently approachable in
practice.

The practical dilemma, however, seems to counterpose what
is, on the one hand, a morally or rationally persuasive ideal
and the impossibility of achieving it in practice. One resolution of the dilemma would seem to be apparent: do the best
you can in the circumstances, even though the ideal norm is unattainable. But the "best possible", falling short of what is
ideally best, is always and to that extent a violation of the
norm. It fails to meet it. The practical argument is that
such "violation" is not deliberate, or in open rejection of
the ideal norm, but in fact is an attempt to act in accordance
with it, within the limits of what is practically feasible.

Now, feasibility connotes limits imposed upon action which
are external and not under the control of the agent. But, in
a practical dilemma of the sort we are considering, practical
constraints also include not merely external limits but also the
demands which practical needs or values place upon the agent.
Thus, the need or demand for the testing of a new drug, to
assure its safety before it is made available for general use,
or to discover its properties or action or side-effects, seems
to be a socially practical imperative. Should it therefore be
put in the balance against the risks and perhaps even against
rights? That is the question which the Prisoners' Dilemma raises,
and it is in this framework of the practical dilemma that I
want to take up the question of the use of prisoners in drug
testing. A final note on the practical dilemma before proceeding.
The alternative resolution (or dissolution) of the dilemma,
other than simply saying "do the best you can", is to question
the moral ideal which is unattainable in practice. Kant's

dictum was "ought implies can"; that is, any viable or rational moral imperative must be one which is practically feasible to realize, for otherwise it remains an abstract piety. But even here, there remains a residue of the dilemma. What one does in fact do is not always, or not often, at the limit of what one can do, where "can" connotes what it is possible to do at the limit. In short, if one argues that one can always do better, then "ought" still posits an ideal not actually realized in practice, although potentially realizable with constant striving at improvement. This tends to be a meliorative approach, in the sense that it proposes the possibility that one's best can always be bettered. Yet in such a formulation, the "best" in the sense of what one ought, at the limit, be able to do, is a limit concept; that is, it can be approached asymptotically, but never finally achieved. On such a reading of "can", "ought" remains the regulative ideal forever just beyond the best we can at any time achieve.

In the context of the Prisoners' Dilemma, this would mean that the ideal of human rights to be observed in the use of prisoners remains at best a limit to be approached, but never reached; and thereby can come to justify a meliorative approach which says, in effect, that although present forms of drug testing in prisons do violate (or fail to fully realize) the human rights of prisoners, these forms can be improved to recognize such rights more fully. These rights then function as the regulative ideal, the "ought" which the "can" strives to achieve. The practical dilemma then remains (residually) in effect; but it is simply taken as a feature of the human condition, to be lived with, even as the attempt is made to progressively narrow the gap between ideal and actuality. This, as we shall see, is one of the alternative "resolutions" of the dilemma, which neither escapes it, nor strictly speaking resolves it at all, but recognizes it as a permanent feature of drug testing in prisons.

There are, as I remarked earlier, two questions concerning both parts of premise (d): (1) are the human rights of prisoners violated in drug testing? and (2) are there medical and social benefits from such testing? Since there would be no dilemma if there were no benefits from such testing, an easy resolution of the dilemma would be to show that the alleged benefits are nil, and that therefore drug testing in prisons is a redundant and unnecessary procedure. I will consider that possibility last, since what concerns us first is what, if anything, constitutes a violation of

human rights in the prison drug-testing context. For if it
can be argued that no such rights are violated, then again
there is no dilemma. I will argue however that there is such
violation, and that it is systemic; i.e. that it is not an
accidental or aberrant feature of such programs , but is
built into their nature. To examine this question, I will
consider, in the first place, what is the ideal or normative
context of human rights, in terms of which one would make
judgments about the treatment or use of prisoners in medical/
pharmaceutical experimental research. In short, what are the
rights we would want to preserve for such experimental subjects?

Since we are speaking of human rights, one way to begin
is to establish the premise that prisoners are human beings.
As simple and obvious as that premise may be, a great deal
follows from it. In the first place, it follows that what is
morally required in the treatment of human beings is equally
required for persons who are prisoners and those who are not.
That is, prisoners have an equal right to be treated with
dignity, with respect for their autonomy, their lives and
their well-being. More specifically, in relation to their
status as subjects for medical experimentation or drug-testing, there are the same requirements for free and informed
consent as have been established for the use of any human
subjects of experimentation. The status of prisoner is
certainly different with respect to civil rights of a certain
kind, to be sure. With imprisonment, as punishment for a
crime of which one has been found guilty, there comes the
loss of specific civil rights, under the law--freedom of
movement, voting, etc. But the loss of these rights is still
compatible with the retention of other civil rights--e.g.,
to own property, to due process under the law, etc.; and
certainly compatible with the retention of those essential
rights which define our humanity. Thus, the loss of certain
civil rights under the law, as punishment for crime, does not
and cannot entail any loss of rights which prisoners have as
human beings. To the extent that such rights are violated,we
may justly complain of inhumane treatment of prisoners, for
it is no part of civil law to deprive any person of those
essential rights which they have qua human beings.

That prisoners retain their human rights is an essential
premise of my argument that these rights are violated in the
present use of prisoners in pharmaceutical Phase I experimentation. For the condition required in such experimentation is

that the subjects give free and informed consent to be put at
risk in such experiments. Any form of coercion which induces
one to act without such freedom, and without an understanding
of the potential hazards therefore violates this condition.
The requirement is clearly and unambiguously set forth in
the two signal documents which concern experimentation with
human subjects, the Nuremberg Code and the Declaration of
Helsinki of the World Medical Association. The language of
the Nuremberg Code states that "the voluntary consent of the
[experimental] subject is absolutely essential," and further,
that the subject should be "so situated as to be able to exercise the power of free choice, without the intervention of
any element of force, fraud, deceit, duress, overreaching, or
other ulterior form of constraint or coercion."[1] The
Declaration of Helsinki likewise requires the "freely-given
informed consent" of the subject (preferably in writing) and
states also that "concern for the interests of the subject
must always prevail over the interests of science and society."[2] It seems clear, therefore that the ideal, normative
case for the human rights of prisoners as experimental subjects poses the moral requirement that the prisoners act as
free agents, with full autonomy in matters of consent to
their use in prison drug-testing programs.

The question I want to raise is whether such voluntary
and uncoerced consent is possible in the prison context. For
the prison context presents several potential forms of constraint or coercion: first, there is the very general situation of duress which prison-life breeds. This is not to say
that this duress is itself a coercion to subject onesself
to experimental testing, but rather that it operates as the
negative background against which the improved conditions of
life as an experimental subject become an inducement. Second,
there is the inducement of money paid for participation in
drug-testing. This is, as I will presently discuss it, a
rather complex matter of coercion, both in the general context
of "doing it for money" as an experimental subject, and in
the specific context of the scale and effect of such monetary
inducement under prison conditions. Third, there is the potential constraint, or inducement that participation in testing
programs may carry with it the reward of being counted in
favor of the prisoner in considerations of parole or length
of sentence, which creates a pressure to take part in such
programs. Beyond these three potential constraints of better
living conditions, money, and improvement of parole chances
or reduction of sentence, there is another aspect of special

discrimination which may also be seen as a constraint, or a
form of involuntary participation in drug-testing. It derives
from the very suitability of prisoners as a testing-population.
What is regarded as a necessary condition for pharmaceutical
experimentation, on statistical grounds, is the availability
of a cloistered, relatively stable and controllable population
of experimental subjects. This is important not only for the
purposes of immediate test-results, but for follow-up studies
as well. Prisoners thus provide such a special population
under constraint (of incarceration for definite, or predictable
periods of time) and available therefore for experimentation
which the normal, non-prison population is not suited for.
(There are, of course, other such cloistered, control populations, e.g. in nunneries, or in some forms of military service,
but these do not concern us here.) One might argue that this
is simply a special opportunity, or a mode of the division of
labor in society, and that it is fortunate that such statistically suitable controlled populations are available. But it
is a statistical consequence of this suitability that the
prison population is in a situation that puts a higher percentage of it at risk in medical and pharmaceutical testing
than is the case for the normal population. And even with a
low probability of risk, if one multiplies it by the number
of participants which is percentagewise higher than is the
case with experimental subjects in the normal population,
the prison population may be seen to be the object of special
discrimination in this regard. Moreover, who constitutes this
prison population? Again, it is statistically skewed with
respect to the normal population, since it is largely black
and poor, in percentages much higher than are representative
of the population as a whole. It is this special population
to which are offered, in the prison context, the inducements
mentioned earlier. Since, in the life of prisoners, better
regime, treatment, food, quarters etc. count for a great
deal; and since, in the economy of prison life, money counts
a great deal, what we have is a situation which is morally
questionable because of the special force of such inducements
for a highly vulnerable group to get them to put themselves
at risk in drug-testing. If such inducements constitute a
form of coercion, as I will argue that they do, then this
constitutes a case of special discrimination against a specific population. The coercion here may be characterized as
a statistical sort of coercion, since it operates not simply
with respect to individual cases of free and informed consent,
but also with respect to the statistical vulnerability of a
whole social group, namely, prisoners who are, to a degree

much greater than the normal population, black and poor.

It has been objected that such inducements as I have mentioned are just that, i.e. inducements, and that therefore this cannot be regarded as a case of coercion. It is, at most, a form of bribery; and bribery, unlike coercion, does not violate the condition of free or voluntary consent of the bribee. One chooses freely to accept a bribe, after all; and therefore, one is held responsible for having accepted it. That is, in general, true. But there is a condition of induce- ment or bribery which it seems to me is coercive, where the special vulnerability or need of the bribee is exploited by the briber, and in which case the offering of a bribe or an inducement may be a morally culpable act, and the accepting of a bribe or an inducement may be seen to involve one of those "ulterior modes of coercion or constraint" which the Nuremberg Code speaks of. Thus, though one may argue that it is not a human right not to be bribed or induced, it never- theless is a human right--namely, the right to choose freely, or to act free from force or coercion--which is at stake when the inducement is such, and one's vulnerability to it is such, that one's consent is obtained under constraint.

I have argued, in another article concerning the use of paid experimental subjects in general, that the sale of the disposition over the use of one's body for experimentation necessarily involves some degree of coercion or constraint, and that it is not a free and voluntary act.[3] I will not repeat the argument here, but its upshot is that putting one- self at risk for payment is coercive, since it is precisely a matter of doing something for money which one would not have voluntarily agreed to otherwise. The analogy may be drawn to wage-labor. Here, it would seem there is a voluntary and informed agreement to exchange a certain portion of one's working time for money, and that coercion can hardly be said to be involved in ordinary work for wages. But this masks a crucial feature of the ordinary work-situation. The worker is not free not to work, for without the wage, he or she cannot live. But then, it may be argued, on these very grounds, that the prisoner is free to refuse to participate in experimentat- ion, since his or her life does not depend on it. I believe that constraint or coercion is not always a matter of life or death, however. Just because of the loss of freedom which is involved in imprisonment, and the constrained and impover- ished mode of existence which this entails, the inducement to better one's living conditions, one's monetary status, or

one's term of imprisonment is no simple inducement, as it
might be in normal conditions outside prison, but is a form
of coercion or constraint which compromises the requirement
for free consent which the Nuremberg Code sees as "absolutely essential."

There is another aspect to such coercion which bears on
the question of exploitation of prisoners in pharmaceutical
testing. I remarked earlier that in offering monetary inducement and superior living conditions to experimental subjects,
the pharmaceutical companies that engage in drug-testing in
prisons are morally culpable in using such inducements to
a specially vulnerable population. In this sense, they are
taking advantage of the special neediness or life-conditions
of the subjects. Moreover, it seems to be the case, _prima
facie_, that the rate at which such experimental subjects in
prisons are paid is exceptionally lower than that which would
have to be paid outside the prisons, to subjects in the normal
population. The immediate conclusion would seem to be that
the drug companies, or the researchers are cleaning up on this
procedure, economically, e.g. paying a dollar a day for what
would cost $40, $50 or even $100 a day in total expenses
outside the prison. In another sense, the State subsidizes
part of the cost of such experimentation by maintaining the
prison population as a pool of experimental subjects. It would
seem then that this is a case of super-exploitation by the
drug companies, given the prospective profits from the sale
of drugs, in contrast to the minimal costs of maintaining
and operating the test-facilities.

There is an interesting counterargument to this, which
bears on the question of coercion. The argument is that
just because ordinary extra-prison monetary amounts are
hugely multiplied in the spare prison economy, payment at
normal rates would provide too great an inducement to the
prisoners, and would therefore tend to be coercive. Thus, in
order to avoid coercion, prisoners are paid at a minimal rate,
so that the pressure to participate in risk-taking experiments
will not be excessive. In some prisons, the "normal" payment
is divided between the reasonably minimal amount which goes
to the individual test-subjects, and the balance which goes
into a general welfare fund, for the benefit of all the prisoners. Thus, the individual prisoner is contributing to the
welfare of the general prison population by taking part in
testing-programs. Now this appears to me to be a reasonable
procedure, in the two respects that it minimizes the coercive

effect of the monetary inducement, and introduces an element
of community in prison life, where each contributes to the
welfare of all. But this is a tricky benefit, in moral terms.
One of the motives in keeping the monetary payment to the
individual prisoner low is not merely to avoid coercion, but
to avoid skewing of the test results. If the inducements of
testing are high, then prisoner-subjects will (and do) tend
to want to continue in the testing situation as long as
possible. They will, in effect, be induced to continue to
put themselves at risk, even to the extent of not reporting
symptoms or ailments in order to stay in the program and to
make the extra bucks. What is telling about such occurrences
is that they point up the extraordinary vulnerability to
inducement of the prison population, and make dramatically
clear how far such inducement goes in the direction of
coercion. Moreover, even where a nominally "normal" rate
of payment is applied, with a portion going into a general
welfare fund for the prisoners, the question arises as to
how such a going rate is determined. The question of exploitation requires some computation of what the "fair market
rate" would be , in the general economy, for putting oneself
at risk in experimental procedures.

Now there is risk involved in many occupations, even
ordinary ones which are not especially regarded as risk-taking
professions. The risks here are part of the job, so to speak.
Especially risky professions, like mining, structural steel
construction, deep-sea-diving, test-piloting, either do or
ought to include the degree of risk in the computation of
payment for such work. But participation in medical or
pharmaceutical experimentation is different in kind from
even such risky professions, not because of the difference
in degrees of risk--it may be larger in some of these profes-
sions--but because of the distinctive nature of such experimentation. Here, the subject is deliberately putting at risk
something which is invaluable and irreplaceable, namely,
one's health, one's body, or even one's life. Though these
are also at risk in other professions, they are incidentally
at risk. The point of the job is not to put them at risk, but
to mine coal, build a skyscraper, test a plane. Here, in drug-
testing, the point of the job is to risk one's health and
body deliberately, to test the safety, or the side-effects
of a drug or a medical procedure. There is, then , a quali-
tatively different intention. The job of the experimental
subject may then be seen to be a special kind of job; and
the condition of free and informed consent in such a situation

seems to me to require more than merely consent to what someone else is going to do to the subject. It seems to require,
in addition, some degree of control over the conditions of
that risk, and some participation in the planning, the review
and the assessment of the results of the procedure itself.
For the consent to be free and rationally informed, the
understanding of what is involved, and the judgment of the
degree of risk, as well as the assessment of the possible
benefits would seem to me to require that the experimental
subjects themselves participate in the phases of the
procedure, not simply as objects to be acted on and used,
but as rational agents. Beyond this, it seems to me that the
assessment of the value of the risk, in monetary terms, is
also part of what falls within the purview of the participating experimental subjects. That is, the rates at which such
experimentation is paid for ought to be subject to negotiation with the prisoners themselves, or with their chosen rep-
resentatives.

Precisely because the present organization of drug-testing in prisons tends to be coercive for all the reasons I
suggested above, it imposes on the autonomy and rationality
of the prisoners, and treats them as less than human. On an
ideal construction of what human rights prisoners ought to
have, if they are to be treated as full human beings, one
would have to grant them, as experimental subjects, some
degree of control over the conditions of their activity.
The condition of being human is the condition of having and
exercisihg one's freedom. Now prisoners are constrained and
coerced in many ways, as prisoners, under the law. That is
a separate matter, however. Whatever violations there may be
of their human rights as prisoners, or even of their civil
rights, as prisoners, is not the specific subject of this
paper. But insofar as they are experimental subjects, the
fact that they are prisoners is not at all germane, because
the experimental procedure is neither a part of their punishment nor a part of their rehabilitation; nor is it any part
of their treatment as prisoners. The separation of these two
things--their status as prisoners and as experimental subjects--
becomes a moral imperative. As experimental subjects, they
may not be treated in any way that distingusihes them as
prisoners, i.e. neither for punishment nor for purposes of
amelioràtion of their lot nor for rehabilitation. Thus, one
may not argue that it is good for prisoners to participate
in drug-testing, because it contributes to the social welfare
and will make them better people. Nor may one argue

that drug-testing programs are better for the prison economy
or provide gainful employment for the prisoners. For none
of these things have to do with the function of the prison,
nor with the purposes of justice, nor with obligations or
responsibilities that the prisoners have, qua prisoners.
We are talking about non-therapeutic drug-testing programs
which are not conducted either for the benefit of the prisoners
or for the benefit of the prison system. Therefore, within
this domain, the prisoner is not a prisoner, but an experimental subject only. As such, he or she is a fully participating
human being , an agent in a procedure which involves putting
his or her health and well-being at risk. In this context,
prisoners , as human beings, have the equal freedom to participate in the decision-making and the control of the experimental procedures, in the review of these procedures, and in
the planning of these procedures.

To the extent that prisoners engaged in drug-testing
are kept from participating in these ways in an activity which
requires their free and informed consent as human beings (and
not in any distinctive way as prisoners, for the reasons given
earlier) to that extent their capacities and rights as human
beings are being infringed. One might argue that non-prisoners
do not at present participate in this way, in medical or
pharmaceutical experimentation; that, as experimental subjects,
whether paid or voluntary, they do not have such rights of
decision-making or review in the experimental procedures.
It is true that they do not, but also, in my view, true that
they should. Still, prisoners are in a different situation.
The non-prisoner is not under the same constraints with respect to civil activity. The prisoner, for example, is not
free to engage in the kind of organizational, legislative
or union activity by means of which the non-prison experimental research subjects can struggle to attain their rights.

Under presently organized forms of drug-testing in
prisons, the human rights of prisoners to exercise the freedom
which they have as experimental subjects , which are entirely
independent of their status as prisoners, are therefore
systematically violated. The violation lies in the coercion
under which the testing is carried out, and such coercion
derives from the nature of the inducements put forth to an
especially vulnerable population. Such coercion, however,
violates the specific requirements for free and informed
consent in experimentation with human subjects.

2. TOWARD AN IMPERFECT RESOLUTION OF THE DILEMMA

In presenting the Prisoners' Dilemma, I counterposed an ideal normative case (for human rights of prisoners) to the practical unfeasibility of attaining the ideal. Nevertheless, I suggested that the ideal case could serve as a regulative norm for improvement, on the grounds that one could always do better than has been done, in ameliorating present conditions. If it is true, as I argued, that coercion is endemic to the prison situation, insofar as present forms of drug-testing exploit the special vulnerability of the prison population, then to that extent, such coercion constitutes a violation of the requirement for free and informed consent, and thus also violates the human rights of the prisoners to be free of coercion in those actions which do not fall under the civil coercion which imprisonment represents. My argument here was that , as experimental subjects, prisoners were equal to non-prisoners, since the situation of drug-testing had absolutely nothing to do with the contexts of punishment or rehabilitation of prisoners, and was not in any way a constituent of prison-functions. Given all this, it would seem that the dilemma is unresolvable, unless drug-testing in prisons can be so reorganized as to be entirely without coercion, by any of the means, overt or covert, which I have reviewed; or else, drug-testing in prisons is given up altogether. Short of such resolutions of the dilemma (by eliminating one or the other of the horns), there is the alternative of doing the best we can to improve things, accepting the dilemma as a condition of life, and hoping to minimize it.

I have suggested how drug-testing may be reorganized, with respect to the participation of prisoners in some degree of control over the procedure, in planning, decision-making and assessment, and also with some means of negotiating the terms of payment. These ameliorative proposals have a practi- cal end of improving the lot of the experimental subjects and lessening the degree of exploitation of the prison population in drug-testing programs. But they have an ideal end as well, realized in this very practice: they are means of extending and exercising the autonomy of the prisoners in the domain where their autonomy is a condition for their human rights--i.e. as experimental subjects, where their status as prisoners is normatively indifferent, and irrelevant.

I do not suppose that even with such changes in the sys-

tem, there will be no more coercion. It will persist, even if
in attenuated form, as long as there exists an especially
vulnerable population of prisoners for whom such drug-testing
programs provide inducements which, by contrast to the conditions of prison life otherwise, are effective in getting the
experimental subjects to put themselves at risk. It also
seems unreasonable, on the other hand, to eliminate a means
by which prisoners can, in fact, improve their lot, even if
temporarily and at the cost of some risk. A meliorative-prac-
tical approach seems to suggest that optimally, what can be
accomplished is some control by the prisoners over the conditions under which they put themselves at risk. Also, a general
change in the social context which produces a disproportionate
percentage of prisoners from among the least advantaged and
most oppressed sections of the population, e.g. the poor and
the blacks, would ameliorate the special discrimination I
spoke of earlier. But these are long-range and complex goals.
Given the persistence of the coercion and exploitation in one
or another degree, does one compromise oneself morally by
seeking such melioration in the face of the continued violation of the ideal norm? Is one coopted into tacitly supporting
a coercive system in trying to improve it?

There are, I think, three alternatives here: first, one
may question an ideal norm which stands beyond practical real-
ization, and reformulate it so that it becomes a feasible
one. Second, one may reinterpret the very notion of an ideal
norm—e.g. of human rights—as regulative, so that its very
function is to serve as a guide, and a goad to improvement
and change in its direction. That is to say, the ideal exists
not beyond practice, but as a practical guide. Third, one
may question the necessity or benefit of drug-testing in
prisons altogether. We have examined the first two possibilities to some extent. Let us consider the third, briefly.

Two questions arise here. First, is the benefit derived
from testing so great that for its sake we should be ready to
live with the dilemma, countenance the persistent violation
of human rights of prisoners, even if to diminishing degrees
with improvements in the organization of testing, and try to
do better? Or is the whole procedure of pharmaceutical Stage
I testing one which could be carried out by means other than
in prisons? Or more sharply still, is the moral problem of
the violation of the human rights of prisoners so serious,
that alternative methods of testing must be found, even if
they are less statistically well-controlled or effective?

Such questions lead us into considerations which up to now have been avoided, namely, cost-benefit considerations, or considerations of the relative utilities of alternative approaches. I will not enter into them here, because I think they are not germane to the problem posed in this paper. Although it is right to try to decrease the risk of drug-testing programs, and although there are clear benefits to be derived from the use of cloistered populations like prisoners in drug-testing, and although the social and medical benefit of the introduction and testing of new drugs is also clear, the best case, short of giving up prison drug-testing altogether, still maintains the dilemma. There are arguments for drug-testing in the population at large, rather than among prisoners; and of course, there are arguments against that. Again, this is not the focus of the present paper. Realistically, it is quite clear that drug-testing in prisons will continue, and that prisoners' human rights in this regard will continue to be violated.

In this regard, it seems to me the only resolution of the Prisoners' Dilemma is an imperfect one: to strive for the greatest improvement possible, to find those practical ameliorative means which will mitigate to the greatest extent possible the exploitative aspects of testing programs, and the violations of the human rights of prisoners; and to live with the dilemma without forgetting it. For our recognition of it keeps us morally sensitive to what might otherwise become acceptable to us.

REFERENCES:

1. The Nuremberg Code, in Trials of War Criminals Before the Military Tribunals Under Control Council Law No. 10, Vol. II, Nuremberg, October 1946-April 1949. Reprinted in T.L. Beaucham and L. Walters, Contemporary Issues in Bioethics, California: Wadsworth, 1978, pp. 404-405
2. Declaration of Helsinki, adopted by 18th World Medical Assembly, Finland, 1964. Reprinted in Beauchamp and Walters, op. cit., pp. 405-407
3. Marx W. Wartofsky, "On Doing it for Money", in Research Involving Prisoners, Appendix to Report and Recommendations, The National Commission for the Protection of Human Subjects of Biomedical and Behavioral Research, DHEW Publication No. (OS) 76-132, Washington, D.C., 1976, pp. 3-1 - 3-24

Troubling Problems in Medical Ethics: The Third
Volume in a Series on Ethics, Humanism, and Medicine: 73-78
© 1981 Alan R. Liss, Inc., 150 Fifth Ave., New York, NY 10011

DRUG TESTING IN PRISONS

Robert J. Levine

Professor of Medicine and Lecturer in
    Pharmacology
Yale University School of Medicine
New Haven, Connecticut

About four or five years ago, I visited Ann Arbor with
the National Commission for the Protection of Human Subjects
of Biomedical and Behavioral Research. Our purpose was to
make a site visit to the Jackson State Prison. We saw a lot
of interesting things there; among other things, we met with
a group of maximum security prisoners who discussed their
research program and their attitudes about it. One of them
said something that stuck with me. He said, "We understand
from your title, Commission for the Protection of Human Research Subjects, that you must be here to protect us from
something. We don't know if you understand that you're in
a place where death at random is a way of life. We have
noticed that the only place that people don't die here is
in the research unit. Just what is it you think you're
protecting us from?" I was impressed with that.

I shall begin with a look at the case that we have been
given to consider. I shall concentrate on some of the things
that seem to me either incorrect or misleading. I shall also
use this case as a springboard for some comments that I
would like to make.

First, some incorrect statements. On the first page we
find a statement that hundreds of dollars a day might be
given to non-prisoner volunteers with the implication that
this would be to induce them to participate in the same sort
of research we are considering today. This is not correct.
In general, volunteers for research are paid according to
customary market factors. Participation in Phase I drug
studies is generally regarded--at least tacitly--as unskil-

led labor. Customarily, subjects are paid approximately the minimum wage, perhaps slightly more. Thus the rate of pay is in the order of magnitude of $25 daily. The estimates of pay scales for prisons that appear in the case study are approximately correct. One is led to wonder then if this motivates drug companies to involve prisoners as subjects simply because they cost less. I don't think so. In fact, although the difference in pay scales is about 10 to 15 fold, this is really a trivial portion of the drug development budget. It's been calculated by people in the drug industry that the salaries to research subjects run somewhat less than one hundredth of 1% of their drug development budget. So I doubt that this differential in pay scales is a powerful motivating factor.

Now, it might seem exploitive to pay prisoners approximately 50 cents to $2.00 daily. This is the pay range for most jobs in prisons. Typically, the pay to the research subjects in the prison is placed slightly above the middle of the range of pay scales in the prison for other jobs. Also, it interests me that in those prisons that have educational programs, the pay to participate in those tends to be slightly below the median for pay to hold jobs in the prison. In general, an agreement is made with the prisoners that if they take pay for educational programs, they are not allowed to simultaneously hold another job. The reason that pay scales for research subjects are set near the middle of the range for jobs in the prison is to avoid what might be considered an undue inducement. If we think these rates of pay are exploitive, and I personally do think they are exploitive, then to be consistent, we must argue that all salaries in a prison are exploitive, and that all salaries in the prison should be commensurate with what is being paid on the outside. Meanwhile, we must acknowledge that we are now exploiting prisoners to make license plates, shoes (as I recall, at Jackson they make shoes) and other such things. And, as I am going to point out shortly, these enterprises are in general substantially more dangerous than Phase I drug studies.

Now, the National Commission for the Protection of Human Subjects of Biomedical and Behavioral Research (I'm going to refer to this as "the Commission"; I am aware that there are many other Commissions, but I would rather not have to repeat its very long title too often), suggested two alternative approaches to dealing with the pay problem in prisons. First, they suggested that sponsors should be required to pay the same amounts of money for prisoner subjects as they pay for non-prisoner subjects. But to avoid the implications of undue inducement, they should give only that amount to the prisoner that would be commensurate with other pay scales within the prison; the remainder of the money should be put into a general fund to be administered by the prisoners to support the welfare, general well-being, or perhaps even health benefits of the prisoners. This is something that was commonly done even before the Commission came along. For example, in the highly publicized Maryland prisoners case, it was established that the average rate of pay for the prisoner-subject was $2 daily; the sponsors of the research paid $10 daily of which 8 went to a general fund for the prisoners' welfare.

The second alternative suggested by the Commission was to hold the difference in escrow and then give it to the prisoner or the prisoner's family after release from the prison. It seems to me that this alternative is really not responsive to the notion of undue inducement, because the individual prisoner-subject still receives the relatively large sum of money.

On page two of the case before us, we find a reference to the work of Zarafonetis and his colleagues, work that was done right here in the Michigan prison system designed to estimate the hazards of drug testing. There is a correct statement that in this population no anti-cancer drugs were studied. This could be construed (as this case is written) to mean that Zarafonetis underestimated the hazards of research in prisons. However, because of the well-known very high toxicities of most anti-cancer agents, Phase I studies of anti-cancer agents are rarely done in normal volunteers, whether they are in or out of prison. In my opinion, Zarafonetis has provided an accurate estimate of the hazards presented to prisoners by participation in drug studies. Let us now consider his data in somewhat more detail in order to develop further perspective on the risks of drug research.

Zarafonetis et al tabulated the adverse consequences of all drug studies conducted in the Michigan prison system over a long period of time. This involved an examination of two-thirds of a million subject-days of involvement in drug studies. They reported on what they called "clinically significant medical events." The definition of such events was very inclusive; almost anything that went wrong was included. They found one "event" for every 26.3 years of subject exposure to drugs--only one thing went wrong every 26.3 years. In the entire study, there was one death; this was a "healthy" prisoner who died of a cerebral hemorrhage in his sleep while taking a placebo. There was only one instance of permanent disability which might have been related to an investigational drug, but clearly could not have been caused by the drug.

Now let us consider the other study to which our case alludes. This is the very extensive study conducted by Cardon and his colleagues for the HEW Secretary's Task Force on Compensation of Injured Research Subjects. They found that 0.1% of the subjects sustained temporary disability. They further reported that less than 0.1% sustained permanent disability. In their report to the Task Force they provided the exact number; it was one case out of 93,339 subjects--approximately 1000th of one percent.

It is correct that in his paper, Cardon distinguished between "therapeutic" and "non-therapeutic" research. But this is something we should never do. In fact, Cardon subsequently has acknowledged that this was an error. Using the distinction between "therapeutic" and "non-therapeutic" research invariably creates confusion. I will come back to that point in just a little while.

But let us first go along with the language that he used in his paper and look at what he then called "therapeutic research." We find that the apparent risks are very substantially higher then they were for "non-therapeutic research." This does not mean anything except that the subjects of "therapeutic research" are sick; they need various forms of therapy to deal with their diseases. These therapeutic modalities produce complications, whether they are established standard therapies or investigational therapies. A comparison of Cardon's data on the complications of "therapeutic research" with other published reports on the hazards of medical therapy and hospitalization suggests that it is less perilous to be a research subject than a patient. The risk of death or disability (physical, psychological, permanent or temporary disability each considered separately) in what Cardon et al called "therapeutic research" was approximately half of what it is for patients receiving

standard medical care in hospitals. I don't mean to say
that it is safer in general to receive investigational
therapies, but there is something about the selection of
subjects and the monitoring process and other special pre-
cautions taken in research that seems to create a much safer
environment.

In the final paragraph of the case study you are asked
to decide whether you would permit "therapeutic research"
involving prisoners; in my view this question does not permit an answer. Research is an enterprise that is designed
to develop generalizable knowledge; by contrast, therapy is
an enterprise that is designed to enhance the well-being of
an individual. There used to be a sloppy habit of calling
the act of administering an investigational drug "therapeutic
research;" various commentators, myself included, have examined and exposed the logical flaws inherent in this: quite
simply, "therapeutic research" is a contradiction in terms.
If you examine carefully any ethical code or set of regulations that relies on the spurious distinction between
"therapeutic research" and "nontherapeutic research" you
will find serious problems. For example, the Declaration
of Helsinki, literally interpreted, requires that all research designed to explore the pathogenesis of a disease
be done either on normal volunteers or on patients who do
not have the disease. To avoid such problems the Commission
repudiated the distinction between "therapeutic" and "nontherapeutic research" and the proposed DHHS and FDA regulations
also have abandoned this distinction. For further discussion
of this issue see (Levine, 1979).

The case study also calls upon you to decide whether
or not you would permit Phase I drug studies to be conducted
in Detroit State Prison. It is worth keeping in mind that
as of this year, these studies are strictly forbidden.by
the regulations of both FDA and DHHS. These regulations
permit research designed to evaluate the safety and efficacy
of practices, both innovative and accepted. Note that this
is not "therapeutic research;" it is research on practices.
Such research may be done only if it can be shown that the
prisoner-subjects are expected to get some direct health-
related benefit from the practice modality that is being
studied. This, of course, can never be the case in Phase I
studies. The regulations forbid all other biomedical research unless it is designed to examine conditions that
particularly affect prisoners as a class; for example, re-

search on hepatitis including vaccine trials is permissible. Also permissible is research on social and psychological problems such as alcoholism, drug addiction, and sexual assaults.

In order to get any good out of discussing the case that is presented to you, I suggest you conduct your discussions as though these regulations did not exist. You might consider whether these regulations are warranted ethically; if not, what alternative guidelines might be more suitable for the conduct of research on prisoners? To this end I think that Professor Wartofsky has provided several arguments that merit consideration.

One final point: It is very easy to challenge the validity of using normal volunteers as subjects for Phase I drug trials regardless of whether the volunteers are imprisoned. It is very difficult to defend this practice on either ethical or scientific grounds. Ethically, while the risks of injury to subjects are of low probability, the benefits to the subjects are always non-existent; thus the personal harm to benefit ratio is always infinity. Scientifically, the data they yield are generally much less relevant to subsequent clinical use of the drug than they would be if subjects were drawn from the population of those having the disease the drug is designed to treat (as is the case in most countries other than the United States). Rather than spending the time allotted to discussion of this case to questioning the ethical and scientific validity of Phase I drug testing on normal volunteers, I suggest that you accept as a given that we live in a society that encourages--in fact, requires--such practices. Given this, are there any reasons that you might wish to exclude prisoners from participation in such programs?

REFERENCE

Levine, R.J. (June, 1979). Clarifying the Concepts of Research Ethics. Hastings Center Report 9(No. 3) 21-26.

**Troubling Problems in Medical Ethics: The Third
Volume in a Series on Ethics, Humanism, and Medicine: 79–89
© 1981 Alan R. Liss, Inc., 150 Fifth Ave., New York, NY 10011**

DRUG TESTING IN PRISONS: THE VIEW FROM INSIDE

Pat Duffy, Jr.
Jackson Prison
Jackson, Michigan

(EDITOR'S NOTE: The following is a minimally edited
transcript of Mr. Duffy's presentation and his subsequent answers to questions from conference participants. Unlike the other speakers, Mr. Duffy has
not had an opportunity to review and revise his
transcript before publication.)

Good morning. I was informed about this seminar about
two days ago, and I was't told what to prepare for except to
come down and look at you and answer a lot of questions that
you might have about testing in a prison. My area of expertise,
of course, is all kinds of criminal acts, how to survive in
Jackson prison (a maximum security facility), how to get
along, how to make money within the prison structure, and
various and sundry other things you only read about in the
newspaper. I have listened to both of the speakers that
preceded me. I agree with some of that they said, and so
what I want to do in the shortest possible time here is to
approach a few things these two gentlemen have kicked out,
and answer your questions, whatever they may be.

First of all, I would like to say that although many of
the facts that they have presented are worthy of your consideration, I don't think either of the gentlemen have done
a long bit in prison. At least they haven't admitted to
that. I've been at Jackson Prison for approximately 7
years, got another 6 or 7 years to go unless the judge in
Detroit takes mercy on me. I've been involved in Phase I
testing at Parke Davis and Upjohn and in fact I'm part-

icipating in a test right now. It's a test on ointments. (I
have both arms wrapped, I can pull it down and let you see
what's happening with the ointments. I went over and asked
the people at Parke Davis and Upjohn and they were very
cooperative.)

First of all you have to understand the philosophy of
prison, and you can't do that unless you've been in prison.
There's a lot of do-gooders that come in and take what we
call the ten dollar tour. The prison officials take them
through, and they say, "Oh, this is maximum security; this
is where we keep the bad guys, and these are the guys that
aren't so bad." People walk through, they walk around and
have a cup of coffee and a stale donut from the mess, and
now they're experts on prisons. They go out and tell all
their friends, "Yeah, I've been to Jackson Prison. I know
what it's all about." But you don't know what it's all
about. You don't have to walk in the yard. You don't have
to have your neck on a ball-bearing so you can see 360°
around so that you can protect your life. You don't know
what its all about to be without phones in prison. You don't
know what it's like to be without visits in prison, to be
without your family, without your friends. You don't know
what it's like to lock up every night at nine before it's
dark outside and get up at six in the morning, and so consequently, the whole spectrum of what goes on in prison -
it's not yours to know. It's my world and it's my friends'
world that are up at Jackson or Marquette or any other
prison in the United States.

The thing of informed consent and free choice as regards
a prisoner's life and the programs we participate in can't
be approached in the context that a person on the street
would use. We make choices in prison. We make our own
choices. We are a very definite breed of person. We know
what we are going to do, why we are going to do it, what the
consequences are, the profit that's involved in it. This is
a big part of prison life and all these are choices that
only we can make. When we go over to Upjohn or Parke Davis
and we volunteer for a test (and that's what it is; they
don't recruit, we volunteer), we are informed as to what the
test is going to involve. In fact, we are given quite a bit
of information about it. We are free to get up and walk
out, say we don't want the test. We can start and quit half
way through or a quarter of the way through. There's to my
mind no coercion involved at all. I can tell them to stuff

it. It's not going to inhibit me from future tests. It's
not going to inhibit me from telling my friends to go over
and volunteer for tests. In fact, Upjohn and Parke Davis,
in the minds of most prisoners, is one of the positive
aspects of life in the prison. Parke Davis and Upjohn are
like an oasis in a desert. You go over there when you want
to hide out a little bit, when you want to talk to some
people from the streets, when you want to talk to people
that are going to treat you half way decent. Now, you may
say, "Well, the doctor said that. He said all of these
things are in the form of bribes - better conditions, etc."
But when you look at prison life, you're looking at something completely different from what you have on the outside,
a completely different society. It's turned around. Out in
the street, when you walk around, you say, "Well, someone
might knock me in the head and take my wallet. Someone may
sneak up on me at night by my car and molest me." And
you're right, someone might do that. But when you are
walking around Jackson Prison, you have 300 jerks up there
that you <u>know</u> have done something wrong. When you look at
the guy next to you, he's in maximum security because he's
already done something. You know he's capable of tearing
your head off at any moment. So, Upjohn and Parke Davis,
far from being coercive, far from being something that would
be a detriment to me or my colleagues up there, is looked on
almost like a chapel. We go to those tests, and it's pure
enjoyment. The little bit of irritation that you might be
exposed to on Phase 1 testing is nothing compared to the
madness that goes on in the yard. So you take yourself a
little vacation and then maybe you can face maybe six or
seven more months in the yard or some of these other programs
that they have in the prison system. Dr. Levine said it's
unskilled labor, being on the tests. That's true. No skill
involved. We present our limbs, they put a little ointment
on, then we lay around and watch television, and we drink
coffee, gamble, swear at one another, whatever convicts do.
What you have to understand is that while the labor itself
is unskilled, convicts are very skilled when it comes to
whimpering and snivelling. We get along real good at that.
If my arms itch, I won't sit there quiet, you know. I go
tell the guy, "Look man, this is killing me. You gotta do
something." We're not bashful at all in that regard.

Also, within the prison system in seven years, from
Upjohn and Parke Davis is probably the only time I've received
a complete physical, and I mean they go over you from head

to toe. I'm sure you all know what's involved in a full
physical. There's some things I was a little sceptical
about, thought maybe the guy was a little freaky, but he's
supposed to know what he's doing. But that's one of the
benefits. About every six months or so you get a physical.
You know your ticker is in halfway decent shape. You know
you're going to be able to hold your own in the yard or
whatever, and a lot of guys like it for that reason. They
like to go over and participate just because of the physicals.
The pay is not commensurate with prison wages; it's better.
The money, if you just want to get down to the basics of how
much you get, I can go lay over at Parke Davis for a day and
they will pay me $20 for a skin test. It takes me a third
of a month to earn $20 on my job, and I'm considered skilled
labor in prison. I know you don't like that but, I'm a tool
and die maker. Four year program, one of the college programs.
The pay for the tests is much better than what's paid in the
prison. There's been talk among the convicts there at
Jackson Prison that at one time Parke Davis and Upjohn did
pay even more for the testing and that the system within
Michigan did not want more money kicked out by the two
facilities because it caused problems within the prison.
The problem that this causes is that if you have money in
your pocket, someone is going to rob you if they can, and if
you don't have money you're going to rob someone else. So,
usually when a guy's got a bit of jingle in his jeans,
everybody knows about it. When I get broke, I know who I'm
gonna borrow from. Prison grapevine is fantastic. You
won't believe it. Ten minutes after I'm back today, probably
sixty guys in the yard will know it and I'll be getting a
thousand questions when I walk out.

Anyway, there's a lot of questions I'd like to answer
concerning the testing; I'd like you to be just as forward
as you want. Before anybody asks me, I'm doing 30-50 years.
That's my sentence, so anybody who had that question on the
tip of their tongue, that's it. Don't ask me what for
because I won't tell you. At this time if anybody has any
questions, I'll be glad to answer.

Q: What do prisoners buy with the money?

A: The prisoners (I'm not used to calling us prisoners) we
have two stores. We have a resident store which sells
coffee, canned goods, all the things you would buy in a
supermarket. We have a resident annex which sells clothes,

television sets, radios, tape decks, tapes, socks, underwear, anything that you might find at K-Marts. Not all of the items, but the approved items that will not constitute a security risk in the prison. The prices are generally what you would pay on the street. I think we get a break on cigarettes and coffee. Anybody that smokes can get cigarettes a little cheaper and coffee maybe a little bit cheaper. Tax is eliminated. We don't pay tax. But those are the items that are available. Shoes can be ordered out of a catalogue - we have one vendor and you can order from that vendor only. If you have visits, your people can send you sneakers and it's limited to that. Basically, that's what the money is spent for, other than gambling, dope, etc.

Q: (Dr. Levine) - When I visited there, I heard that a lot of people think that the black prisoners are especially exploited. When I visited there, the black prisoners told us that two thirds of the prisoners there were black and yet only one third of the research subjects were black. They said that was because the white people are in control of the subject selection, white prisoners and white guards, and they discriminate against the blacks. They don't let them be research subjects. Is that still the case?

A: Okay, the testing that is done naturally is picked by Parke Davis and Upjohn. The prison, the guards, and the officers up front at the control center, the lieutenants, the captains, the warden, and so on, really have nothing to do with the subjects that are picked for testing. The only time that they will intervene on a test is if one of the subjects constitutes a security risk. They give a list, and it says "X amount of subjects", usually name, number and lock, are on that list. The list is screened, and they may send a memo back to Parke Davis or Upjohn saying that this man cannot participate on the test because he constitutes a security risk for a certain reason. We don't want him over there at this time. The prison population is predominantly black. Seventy percent of Jackson Prison in the maximum security area, the inside, the central complex, is black. Consequently, it's the whites, the Chicanos, and the Indians who are the minorities in Jackson Prison. The black population by and large runs things in the North Yard, the South Yard, the gymnasium, etc. Most of the workers, the guys that work over at Parke Davis and Upjohn are black, the ones that do all maintenance over there, etc. I couldn't get a job at Parke Davis if I wanted one, and it's one of the

better paying jobs in the institution. I wouldn't be able
to say and I could't say whether or not the choice is pre-
judiced. It well may be. But most of the black guys I know
have participated on the studies, and you've got one of them
in the case report, the one with the messed up head. He's
a good friend of mine. The tests that they can participate
on, they participate on. Usually, like they have one
coming up now on cough syrup - they'll be participating on
that test. The one that I'm on, because of the skin pigment-
ation, they can't test with black subjects. So I think it's
really determined by the test. My experience with the
people at Parke Davis and Upjohn is that they don't exhibit
to my mind too much prejudice. They seem to me like they
are pretty open and accommodating to anybody that comes
over.

Q: How do you know about a project that is coming up? How
are you included?

A: Grapevine. A lot of times we know about a test before
the guys that work over there. There's guys - they have
people working at the facilities in Kalamazoo and they'll
come in the yard and say, "Hey, there's a new hair test
coming down. It's a 120 day walk-in." And the guys'll be
in the block shaving their head bald to get on the test.
Ususally the test that you are going to volunteer for is
determined by how much money is involved or a lay-in. The
guys like to lay-in. The test that I'm on is called a walk-
in test. I go over three times a week, you know, and they
read the patches on my arms and they determine whether or not
the ointment is helping it. They put another patch on, or
they say 24 hours off, and I split. The guys like the ones
where they can go over and put their legs up and drink
coffee and watch color television, you know, all that kind
of thing. If you can get out of the mainstream of the
prison population for a while, that's what you do, and
that's what Parke Davis and Upjohn offer.

Q: So that when you are in treatment, do you feel like you
have more peace of mind then when you are out in the yard?
Do you feel more relaxed?

A: Generally you are over there with other convicts, you
know. I could get offed in one of the facilities just as
well as I could get knocked over in the yard. I ain't felt
safe in seven years. But doing time in prison, you know, is

tough, and it's hard when you come out of prison to get rid
of that facade. You can be an arch coward in the joint, but
don't let anybody know it, because as soon as they know it,
then you can be exploited. That's why young guys coming in,
they have rough times. They're all smooth faced, you know,
when they come in. "Wow, look at this, I'm at the Big
House," you know. Yeah, we classify a young guy as a rabbit.
A guy that's been there a while, he's a bear or a fox.
Foxes, they trick the rabbit into doing what they want; the
bear just beats him to his knees and makes him do what he
wants. Everything has a name, everything has a purpose in
the prison, in the yard, whatever. So put on the mask that
you need to survive, because prison is about survival.
That's what it's about. I mean, look at the context of what
you've heard this morning and say, "Well, Parke Davis and
Upjohn are coercive, because these guys, they go collect
their wits over there. They get theirself back together."
But, hey, to my mind they've probably saved more lives by
just being there for guys to escape into than all their
testing's done. You may question the value of saving convicts,
I don't know. Maybe you'd say, "Let 'em off one another."

Q: From time to time we hear stories from word of mouth or
the newspaper that prisoners in Jackson are contemplating
bringing a suit in some court or another in order to assure
that drug testing continues in prison. Is there a suit in
process now?

A: Yes, sir.

Q: Are you involved in it?

A: I'm not personally involved in it. You might think I
don't want to cop out with it. There are probably two or
three suits that are pending or going to be submitted in
regards to the research that is going on at Jackson Prison
and other facilities. The prisoners don't want it taken
out of prison. In that particular context, I'm saying you
people, the people in courts, in the Federal system, are not
asking us what we want. They are making the choice. Some
prisoners see the testing as a form of repaying their debt
to society.

Q: That was the other question I was tempted to ask. We
are often told by people who write about prison research and
other kinds of research that one of the motivations of

prisoners is altruism and not only the money and the better
conditions. Do you feel that? Do your fellow prisoners feel
that?

A: I think it depends on what game the guy is playing at
the particular time. Some guys run into prison and pick up
a Bible, you know. They might have been real monsters on
the street, but they turn into Oral Roberts when they get in
prison. Everytime you pass a guy, you know, he's sticking
pamphlets in your pockets, you know, you want to smack him
up side the head, you know. The testing program is probably
in some cases used for that. I've heard guys say, "Well,
hey, if this will help somebody I'll do it." It all depends
on what kind of game you are playing.

Q: Who owns the buildings in which the experiments are
done?

A: Maybe I should clarify. The two prettiest buildings
inside the complex are Parke Davis and Upjohn. They build
the buildings and they maintain the buildings, but they are
the property of the state. They were given to the state by
each company, and the state rents them back. It is my
understanding that each building was given to the state and
then rented by the state back to the company for a dollar
for 99 years or something like that. The buildings are well
maintained. They are the newest buildings in the central
complex. Jackson, or the State Prison of Southern Michigan,
as the employees like to call it, is a pretty old facility,
and those are the two newest buildings, and maybe that's
another reason guys like to go over there.

Q: Are there people who just aren't interested in this
testing; and if not, why not?

A: Most of them. I think most of the population inside
Jackson Prison does not want to be involved in the testing.
Convicts have very defined ways of thinking. They are
either for something or against it. Guys out there, you
know, they'll see you with patches on your arms and they'll
say, "Man, you're over there getting cancer," and "Stay away
from me," all that kind of thing. And you try to tell them,
"No, no, I'm on a test with ointment." "No, don't tell me
that man, your arms gonna disappear tomorrow." You know,
they've made up their minds they will never go on a test at
Parke Davis or Upjohn, never. There are others who are saying,

"Hey, who do I see?" But the ratio is probably a vast
number among the prisoners who do not participate by choice
as opposed to those that go over and say they'd like to get
in on this.

Q: Do you know if anybody has ever studied reactions of
prisoners after they have left prison? In other words, they
say they like it and are treated well, but has anyone followed
them and seen whether a year later or two years after they've
been out, that they are sorry they did it or whether they'd
do the same thing again were they not prisoners.

A: I doubt you could catch most guys when they get out. A
lot of them come back two or three times, you know. To my
knowledge, there's not been any follow up on the research
that's been done in these two facilities. Of course, I
can't be positive because I've never asked that question
myself. I have heard guys in the test as recently as a week
ago say, "This is alright. I'd like to do this on the
street. It beats working."

Q: How seriously do you consider the information that is
provided for you at the time before you sign up for these
tests?

A: Let me explain the procedure briefly. We go into a
room that's maybe this size, maybe a little smaller. They
have chairs set up. They pass out literature. For those of
us that can read that's wonderful. There are some guys on
the tests that seriously speaking read at maybe a third or
fourth grade level. I don't know if they understand what
they read, and I'm sure that because of that fact, Parke
Davis and Upjohn have provided that a man that works for the
company comes out and he reads verbatim what's on the sheet.
We all sit there, you know, all excited, waiting. But you
wait for one thing. How much? That's the main thing you
want to hear. If he doesn't say that quick, somebody asks,
"What does this test pay, man?" He then tells you what is
going to happen on the study. "We're going to shave your
arms and we're gonna irritate four patches (on this particular test I'm on) with a 5% solution of Tide soap. The
patches will be on for 48 hours. We will remove them. Then
we will apply ointment. We will take the patches off in 48
hours and see what the effect of the medication is." He
goes through as well as he can what is going to happen
throughout the test. The particular one I'm on is for 39

days, you know, and then he asks if there are any questions.
He asks if anybody does not understand the test. He asks if
anybody wants to eliminate theirself from the test. And in
my experience that has been the procedure throughout the
testing at Parke Davis and Upjohn.

Q: I'm wondering how accurate you think these tests are.
How often might a prisoner lie about the results for whatever
reason so that the final result of the test is unreliable?

A: You're given certain instructions when you're on a test.
I can personally testify to the fact that guys do not always
follow the instructions. For instance, patches; they'll
take them off. They'll look. Convicts are very much like
chimpanzees. They'll ask, "Why is it itching? What's that
bump?" Mind, what I'm saying is all general. All convicts
are not like that. It's something that sets you apart in
the prison population. A lot of guys, I would imagine, they
go in and they wash the medication off. I don't know, maybe
they get some kind of thrill from that. It's a good faith
thing. They say, "We're gonna wrap your arms up" or "We
want you to take this cough medicine three times a day" and
they expect you to do that. Some of the guys they do it
religiously because they think that if they don't, they'll
be found out through their urine sample. Some guys they
dump it down the drain. I've heard them say they do. So I
think you have to really screen the individuals that you are
testing. Possibly that is one of the failings of the program.
Individuals are not really screened that thoroughly. The
results of the tests are Greek to me. I wouldn't know. If
I go in and this guy says the ointment's working, I'll
believe him, because I haven't any medical background. I
know how to put a bandage on my nose if I cut it, or something
like that, but that's about it.

Q; Are you aware of the risk? Do they inform you of the
risks, and have you ever refused an experiment? If not,
where would you draw the line? Where would you in fact
refuse?

A: I'll answer the last part first. I will not take anything
internally. That's where I draw the line. I'm not swallowing
anything that Parke Davis or Upjohn gives me, or anyone
else, for that matter. In fact, when I go to the infirmary,
I don't want to swallow anything they give me, either. And
the worst place to swallow anything is in the mess hall.

So, would you restate the first part of your question?

Q: Do they inform you of the risks?

A: Always. You always know what the risk is. And in Phase
I testing, and I think these two gentlemen covered it pretty
thoroughly, the risk is minimal. I'm probably experiencing
right now on a Phase I test the most severe reaction that
anyone's ever experienced, and it's not from the medication,
it's from the tape.

Q: You have refused tests, then?

A: I have refused tests when they involved any medication
internally. And that includes cough syrup or cough drops;
anything that I gotta put in my gib and swallow. No, it's
not happening.

Troubling Problems in Medical Ethics: The Third
Volume in a Series on Ethics, Humanism, and Medicine: 91-93
© **1981 Alan R. Liss, Inc., 150 Fifth Ave., New York, NY 10011**

DISCUSSION SUMMARY: DRUG TESTING IN PRISONS

Laurie Winkelman
Assistant Program Director, CEHM
University of Michigan
Ann Arbor, Michigan

The majority of the discussants were in favor of allowing
Phase I drug testing in Detroit State Prison. Supporters
of prison experimentation argued that it is within the human
rights of the prisoner to participate in such experiments
and that denying such rights would be an act of paternalism,
and misdirected at that. One sociology student commented,
"Often people with the best of intentions, but who have
never been inside a prison, think they know what is best
for convicts." A professor of law added, "Participation in
experiments gives the prisoner opportunities to make choices
and achieve a sense of purpose." The discussants recognized
that experimentation is regarded by some prisoners as a way
to repay their debt to society, alleviate their guilt, and
achieve feelings of altruism and self-respect. Thus, participation in drug experiments has the potential for satis-
fying human needs.

Opponents of drug experimentation in prisons began
their argument with the contention that prisons are inherently
coercive. They went on to state that the existence of
experimentation creates additional social and financial
pressures on prisoners. Some opponents suggested that the
prisoners think that whether they participate in the experiments influences their parole and their treatment by prison
and medical staff, even though they are told this is untrue.
It was also suggested that the buildings where the experiments take place are more pleasant and safe than the prison
yard. Financial pressures were seen to include the needs of
the prisoners to support their families, to pay legal bills,
and to be monetarily prepared for release from prison.

Possession of money was also deemed necessary to purchase items while in prison since only bare necessities are provided to prisoners. The opponents of experimentation also pointed out that convicts rarely participate in such experiments before coming to or after leaving the prison.

Support for the chemotherapeutic agent study was significantly less unanimous than for the study of the anti-epileptic drug. Those who supported testing the chemotherapeutic agent maintained that the study was for the good of society and needed to be done. Some added that the prison provided a more controlled environment for the study than could be achieved in the outside world. This argument was furthered by one medical student's statement that "If this drug is inappropriately released on the market because of a study that did not have a controlled environment, the entire population of the nation may be subjected to a much greater risk than if the study is performed in the prison setting."

Some of those who opposed testing the chemotherapeutic agent felt that anti-cancer drugs are not needed badly enough to put healthy persons at risk. One person asked, "If the chances of damage to one's health are so small, why don't doctors volunteer to be subjects?" Other discussants felt that too much research is mundane and scientifically insignificant. Other reasons given for disapproving of testing the chemotherapeutic agent were that other countries prohibit experimentation in prisons, that prisoners would bear a disproportionate share of the risk as compared to the general population in such studies, and that prison experimentation constitutes discrimination against minority groups who comprise a large percentage of the prison population.

Further discussion focused upon means of noncoercive compensation in prison settings. A consensus was reached that each prisoner should be paid an amount consistent with prison wages and that an additional amount should be put in a general fund for the prisoners. It was also agreed that the sum of the two payments should still be less than that paid a nonprisoner subject. In reaching these decisions, it was argued that the possession of money by the prisoners tends to reduce hostility, violence, and crime among the prisoners. One philosopher suggested that monetary rewards that buy luxuries rather than necessities do not constitute duress, although some discussants held that inducement in

the outside world could constitute coercion in the prison
setting. A social worker concluded, "If we are worried
about protecting free choice we have to recognize that many of
our life choices both in and out of prison are based on
certain levels of social coercion. The question is where
we draw the line."

**Troubling Problems in Medical Ethics: The Third
Volume in a Series on Ethics, Humanism, and Medicine: 95–96
© 1981 Alan R. Liss, Inc., 150 Fifth Ave., New York, NY 10011**

INTRODUCTION: TREATING CHILDREN WITHOUT PARENTAL CONSENT

Rachel Lipson
Program Director, CEHM
University of Michigan
Ann Arbor, Michigan

The critical illness of a young child places his parents
under tremendous pressure. In addition to the great economic
and emotional burdens engendered by any family member's
illness, they must deal with the unique stress of caring for
a sick child. It is extremely difficult to decide how much
to tell a dying child about his disease, and perhaps it is
equally difficult to force a child to undergo uncomfortable
or painful treatments. Parents, however, are the legal
guardians of their child and in this capacity they must give
informed consent before their child can undergo medical
therapy. They must therefore face these problems and resolve
them rationally.

Few would deny parents the right to refuse treatment
for themselves, but if parents refuse to allow their ill
child to undergo therapy, many ethical and legal questions
arise. What should be done if parents refuse life-saving or
life-prolonging therapy for their child? To what extent
should an older child be consulted about his medical care?
Should a panel of physicians, or a judge, be called upon to
decide what is best for the child and to replace the parents
as legal guardians in such cases? The physician may be torn
between his legal obligation to the parents, who have the
authority to give (or refuse) consent to medical care for
their child, and his moral obligation to the child, who in
the doctor's opinion needs the therapy.

Dr. Relman sets forth several general principles. He
states that the doctor's primary obligation is to his patient
(in this case the child), but warns that the physician must

consider the effects of treatment on the child's family as
well. An antagonistic relationship in the home may also
harm the child. Dr. Relman goes on to consider the notion
of informed consent, saying that the patient should be
informed to the degree he desires. (Relman notes that the
good physician learns to judge what his patient is willing
to hear.) Relman also points out that although the adolescent may be able to make his own decisions, he nevertheless
lacks the legal authority to do so. In these situations,
Relman feels that the physician must obtain consent from the
child (to whatever extent possible) as well as from the
parents. How much say the child should be given depends on
the degree of maturity that the physician judges him to
have.

Finally, Dr. Relman proposes that parents do have the
right, as consenting adults, to refuse treatment for themselves, but they do not necessarily have such a right for
their child who needs treatment. The injustice of denying a
child needed medical care because of his parents' whims must
be avoided at all costs, even if this requires the use of
the imperfect (as Professor Burt points out) legal system.

Professor Burt questions the usefulness of the courts
in cases such as the one presented for this topic because
of the problems inherent in our legal system. He claims
that the biases created by an adversarial due process make
it an inappropriate vehicle for making decisions when
parents may not be acting in their child's best interests.
Burt also points out that the system is often used by those
who want judges to assume the responsibility for making
decisions that the interested parties are themselves afraid
to make. A process by which the parents shirk responsibility for their child seems unlikely to lead to a decision
in the best interests of all those concerned. Burt proposes instead a system of rules to be followed in cases in
which parents and physician disagree about what must be done
in the treatment of a child.

Finally, it should be noted that in his original talk
Professor Burt outlined criteria that should be met before
legal action is considered by the physician. These included
imminent risk to the child's life, and a treatment that
offers near certain cure with minimal side effects. These
comments are not included in Professor Burt's official
manuscript but are referred to in Dr. Relman's paper.

**Troubling Problems in Medical Ethics: The Third
Volume in a Series on Ethics, Humanism, and Medicine: 97–99**
© **1981 Alan R. Liss, Inc., 150 Fifth Ave., New York, NY 10011**

TREATING CHILDREN WITHOUT PARENTAL CONSENT

CASE FOR DISCUSSION

Mr. and Mrs. Smith were very worried. When fourteen
year old Bobby had developed a high fever for the fourth
time in two months, they had assumed that his flu had returned.
Now the doctor was telling them that Bobby had cancer. Dr.
Springer, the hematologist to whom the Smiths had been
referred, explained that acute T cell lymphocytic leukemia
was a cancer of the white blood cells, fatal without treatment. Chemotherapy, however, would offer the child a
significant chance of survival, for 90% of children treated
for the disease are in remission after one year. Dr. Springer
further explained that remission is a period during which
symptoms of the disease are absent and doctors are unable to
detect the disease. This, however, does not mean that the
disease is gone, he cautioned. In fact, only 50% of those
children who undergo chemotherapy survive beyond four years,
but almost all of these are permanently cured. He also
warned that Bobby's age might count against his survival as
most survivors of this disease are much younger and have a
different type of leukemia.

Mrs. Smith wanted to know what would be involved in
chemotherapy and whether it would be uncomfortable for her
son. The doctor explained that the treatment, which would
last for three years, would involve giving Bobby a number of
different drugs in various combinations and in various forms
(i.e., by injection, intravenously, orally). While some
discomfort was associated with the various injections, the
doctor felt that the major side effects would be more uncomfortable. These side effects included loss of hair, loss of
appetite, nausea, joint pains, sleepiness, and headaches.

Frightened but hopeful, Mr. and Mrs. Smith consented to treatment.

After a month, Dr. Springer informed Mr. and Mrs. Smith that Bobby was in remission. Mrs. Smith questioned whether this meant that the boy could stop taking his medicine. The medicine made him sick, she explained, and she hated bringing him to the hospital for his injections so much that she had nightmares before each visit. Dr. Springer once again explained that remission did not mean cure and that the boy had to continue on the therapy. So Bobby underwent special radiation treatment to eradicate cancer cells in his brain and was then put on a program of intermittent low dosage chemotherapy to keep him in remission, as is common procedure in these cases.

Sixteen months later the Smiths did not arrive for their scheduled appointment. Dr. Springer called them to find out what had happened. Mr. Smith explained that he and his wife had decided, along with Bobby, to discontinue Bobby's chemotherapy. The side effects had become intolerable, he explained. The Smiths realized that chemotherapy had gotten Bobby to this stage of remission and had kept him there, but they noted that the disease was almost gone. For this reason, they felt that nutritional therapy involving a special diet was good enough to maintain Bobby in his state of remission. (A friend's uncle who had had cancer and was treated with the diet was still alive and doing quite well.) Dr. Springer tried to convince Mr. Smith of the dangers of discontinuing Bobby's treatment. Mr. Smith thanked the doctor for his concern but said that they had already made their decision. He allowed Dr. Springer to speak briefly with Bobby who confirmed what Mr. Smith said and seemed sure of what he was saying.

Dr. Springer telephoned the Smiths several times over the following two months. Each time they reported that Bobby was doing well on megavitamins and a natural diet. They continued to be adamantly opposed to further chemotherapy, even if Bobby started getting sick again.

At this point, Dr. Springer thinks it unlikely that Bobby can maintain permanent remission without further chemotherapy. He is concerned about Bobby's health and about the ethical implications of allowing Mr. and Mrs. Smith, who mean well but are ignorant of medicine, to decide to refuse Bobby's treatment. Dr. Springer knows how lucky Bobby has been so far, but he wonders if such luck can persist. Based on his reading, he estimates only a 20% chance of cure if Bobby has no further treatment. However, there are no good studies and he is very uncertain of this. Colleagues he consults differ widely in their estimates. He wonders if he ought to get a court order for treatment. On the other hand, he knows how traumatic this might be for the Smith family and wonders if he ought to mind his own business.

Should Dr. Springer go to court? Should he have gone to court when treatment was first refused? Would your decision be different if Bobby were four? Twenty-four? If Mrs. Smith were a doctor? If Bobby were symptomatic again?

(Case prepared by Rachel Lipson and Marc D. Basson.)

Troubling Problems in Medical Ethics: The Third
Volume in a Series on Ethics, Humanism, and Medicine: 101–108
© 1981 Alan R. Liss, Inc., 150 Fifth Ave., New York, NY 10011

TREATING CHILDREN WITHOUT PARENTAL CONSENT

Robert A. Burt

Yale Law School

New Haven, Connecticut

There is a strong tradition in our society that
parents' wishes in rearing their children should be given
great deference. The idea that parents have "rights" in
their children is one way to state this tradition. This
locution these days, however, has a hollow ring, as if it
connotes that children are property rather than persons
and that the concept of parental rights is equivalent to
the idea of chattel slavery. But there is another way to
state the underlying principle of parental rights consistent
with the contemporary individualistic perspective that
demands equal respect for all persons, including respect
for children as persons. From a psychological perspective,
general social deference to parents' wishes in child-
rearing can be seen as the best way to ensure that most
children come into full flowering as individuals. This
social deference, that is, would both acknowledge and
reinforce the intense emotional involvement parents and
children typically have, and must have in order to create
the individualistic adult personality style prized by
this society generally. (This is, in effect, the heart
of the psychoanalytically based argument advanced by
Joseph Goldstein, Anna Freud and Albert Solnit in their
influential books Beyond and Before the Best Interests
of the Child.)

From this psychological perspective, there is no conflict between the idea that every child should be protected
by society in developing the fullest expression of his or
her individual capacities and the idea that society should
defer to parents' decisions in child-rearing. Children

don't spring full-blown into adulthood, some adults must make decisions for them for a considerable time and -- so the argument goes -- outsiders to the child-parent relationship (whether a behavioral expert or a judge or both) cannot forcibly intervene in that relationship without creating excessive risks of psychological harm to the child.

There are, however, some circumstances where it is simply not plausible to argue that this happy concordance of interest exists between parent and child. Child abuse -- brutal parental beatings of young children, for example -- is one such obvious circumstance. In such a case, to use lawyers' language, there is a conflict of interest between parent and child. There is also a conflict of principle on the question of social deference to parental wishes regarding their children; the general rule may be that parents' wishes are generally respected, but child abuse appears an obviously compelling exception to that rule. And using lawyers' language readily leads to invoking lawyers' solutions. Once a potential conflict of interest has been identified between parent and child, and a corresponding conflict among principles also suggested, the standard lawyerly response is to conduct a hearing -- an adversary hearing with each conflicting interest and principle represented by an attorney, and with the responsibility for resolving the conflict vested in a judge. This is what lawyers call the "adversarial due process" model for dispute resolution.

This adversarial due process model has become quite popular among people who consider themselves advocates for children's rights. These people see conflict or potential conflict between parents and children in an increasing number of matters, and argue that these matters should be proceduralized and judicialized. I want to focus in this presentation on the question of parents' medical care decisions, but it is important at the outset to see that current efforts to bring these decisions increasingly into legal fora are part of a general contemporary ideology regarding parent-child conflict. Regarding medical care issues specifically, there are two different circumstances where some people currently argue for judicial recourse: (1) where parents want some medical intervention for their child that others -- perhaps medical professionals, perhaps lawyers -- would oppose; and (2) where parents refuse some

medical intervention that someone else would favor. In
this presentation, I will spend most time discussing the
first circumstance -- where parents want an intervention -- but the considerations I will set out should
have equal applicability to the latter circumstance, as
I will briefly suggest at the end of these remarks.

Three specific situations where parents want medical
interventions opposed by others have been much debated in
the literature and before courts in recent years:

> (1) Parents want to sterilize their severely
>   retarded child;
>
> (2) Parents want to donate one child's kidney
>   to his sibling;
>
> (3) Parents want to place their child in a
>   psychiatric hospital.

For each of these situations, many child advocates
have argued and some courts have decided that parents are
not free to act on their own judgment but that lawyers
must be involved, including the appointment of a lawyer
to represent the child whether or not the child requests
such representation, and that a judge should ultimately
decide whether the parents' wishes should be respected.
Just last year the United States Supreme Court addressed
this issue regarding psychiatric hospitalization
(Parham v. J.R., 99 Sup.Ct. 2493 (1979)); it overruled the
lower court's decision that a judicial hearing was constitutionally required to protect the child's interests.
This Supreme Court decision perhaps will slow the impetus
for lawyers to conceive all manner of parent-child conflict (in medical care or generally) in the adversarial
due process model. But the impetus remains strong nonetheless. For childrens' psychiatric hospitalization,
several state laws now require judicial hearings (notwith-
standing that the Supreme Court has ruled that such
hearings are not constitutionally required), and for
sterilization and kidney donation questions, judicial
proceedings have now become the norm in state laws.

I want to raise some questions about this norm --
this instinctive lawyerly reliance on the due process
model in parent-child conflicts. In this context, I think

the model will not help matters and may even make difficult problems more difficult. There are occasions when parental decisions regarding children should be overruled. But I believe that individual case-by-case hearings before a judge is not a good way -- and perhaps is even the worst way -- to carry out this overruling. I suspect that individualized hearings will distort rather than clarify the issues at stake; I suspect that, no matter what formal procedural checks are devised, the judge will inevitably apply his or her personal biases that will have no necessary connection to the child's interest, the parents' interests or some general social interest. Where parents' decisions must be overruled to protect children, I would not rely on individualized hearings but instead would attempt always to find an alternative regulatory technique.

Let me illustrate the choice between individualized hearings and alternative techniques in the context of sterilization decisions for retarded children. The due process model advocates say, "If parents want to sterilize their mentally retarded children, let them convince a judge after full adversarial hearing." But think for a minute about what would take place at this hearing. Think about the likely impact, for example, of the children's retardation on the judge. How much experience has the typical judge had in dealing with mentally retarded persons? What kinds of attitudes towards mentally retarded people are likely to be percolating in the judge's mind, even if (or perhaps particularly if) he or she has had consider-able experience with such people? What assurances are possible that the judge does not share the common social impulse to diminish the individual worth of those afflicted with mental retardation?

It is difficult to admit and to examine these im-pulses in any setting. But I think it is especially difficult to acknowledge these impulses in the stylized adversarial setting of the courtroom. All of the various legalistic procedures feed the pretense that these feelings are not really operative, that the judge is "impartial" because he has no obvious personal stake in the decision, that the lawyers are "rational" because they speak fluently about balancing this factor against that without admitting how confusing and emotion-laden the sterilization question may be for them as well as for parents and children. The rationalistic tenor of the due process proceeding does not

banish darker impulses so much as it drives them under-
ground where they can silently persist in dominating
decision-making by everyone -- parents, lawyers and judges.

There are reasons to believe that fear and prejudice
regarding the sexuality of mentally retarded persons will
inappropriately distort parents' decisions regarding
sterilization. (See J. Gliedman and W. Roth, The Un-
expected Minority: Handicapped Children in America (1980)
(App. 2: "The Sexuality of the Severely Disabled").) But
it is too glib to assume that these fears and prejudices
will be dispelled in adversarial judicial hearings.

Rather than pretend that such hearings can be
adequately protective of all children's interests, I think
we should force ourselves either to forbid all sterilization of children for birth control purposes or to permit
parents to decide for such sterilization without any
judicial supervision. A rule forbidding all sterilization
might appear excessively harsh and restrictive in some
circumstances. Someone can always identify special
situations that appear to demand exceptional treatment.
Lawyers are particularly adept at finding hypothetical
special problems in general rules and are equally skilled
in suggesting that these case-by-case exceptions can be
identified as easily by lawyers and judges in actual cases.
But I believe that there is considerable slippage between
the hypothetical formulation of an exception and its
identification in actual cases, particularly when the
question is heavily freighted with confusing emotional
overtones. It is true that a general rule forbidding or
permitting parents to authorize their child's sterilization
would prompt abuses in some individual cases. But I
believe it is more honest to admit that individualized
hearings will not adequately protect against abuse and
that any general rule-making on this question should begin
with the premise that no perfect abuse-free mechanism is
possible. From this honest admission, I think it is more
likely that we as a society will focus attention on the
truly relevant considerations.

For sterilization, those considerations include the
availability of alternative but reversible birth control
techniques and their safety and efficacy as compared to
sterilization. It may be that none of the alternatives
to sterilization is as safe or efficacious. On the other

hand, because these other techniques are reversible, they
do appear to answer the concern that parents might inappropriately sterilize mentally retarded children who
could develop adequate parenting capacities by adulthood.
If we hold to the discipline I would impose -- that our
only regulatory options are forbidding or permitting all
sterilization of minors -- we would be forced to choose
between these two unattractive, even incommensurable
options of harming some children by withholding sterilization but subjecting them to less safe or efficacious
birth control methods and harming other children by subjecting them to inappropriate sterilization.

At this point in the argument, the due process model
advocates offer an apparently attractive way out of this
decisional dilemma so that the hard choice of harming some
children to help others seems to vanish. But this is an
illusion -- as much as the possibility of "unbiassed, impartial decisionmaking" on this question by lawyers and
judges is an illusion. This is another reason that the
due process model is so dangerous -- because it is so
seductive. This model of decision-making tells us what
we want fervently to believe; the model appears to refute
the detestable propositions that every social choice
inevitably harms someone, that perfectly harmonious
"justice" is not attainable in this world.

Perhaps it is too difficult to surrender this particular illusion; perhaps I am wrong in thinking that
better social decision-making on behalf of the interests
of children generally would result from this kind of rueful
honesty about the inevitable imperfections in our world.
But consider another illustration regarding parental
medical decisions for children -- kidney donations between
siblings. The law's response to this technological
possibility has been adamant: a judicial hearing is
required to ensure that the parents' decision is in the
donor child's "best interest." (See, for example, Hart v.
Brown, 29 Conn. Sup. 368 (1972)). But what wisdom can
a judge really bring to bear on this question? It may
be that judges' impulses to ratify parents' decisions will
be quite strong in these proceedings and that little harm
will result; and it may be that most parents will authorize
such donation and little harm to the donor child, and
much potential benefit to the donee, will result. And,
finally, it may be that judges' pro forma participation

in these decisions will soothe everyone's irrational, excessive fears about the operation itself and the possibility
that one child has been callously used as a provider of
"spare parts" for another, more favored child. (See the
thoughtful observations by a psychiatrist who participated
in such a judicial proceeding, M. Lewis, "Kidney Donation
by a 7-Year-Old Identical Twin," Journal of Child Psychiatry 13:221 (1974).)

But this is not the avowed purpose of these hearings.
If we are unwilling to admit this true purpose, because
we are unwilling to admit our general misgivings about the
procedure's technical or ethical aspects, then I worry
about the extent to which this hearing will disguise
genuine concerns from all participants, so that once again
children's interests will not be adequately served. For
kidney donation, as for sterilization, I would prefer the
discipline of choosing between a social rule that forbade
or permitted all parental decisions without any case-by-
case judicial supervision. For myself, I would opt for a
rule permitting parental decisions regarding kidney
donations and forbidding such decisions for sterilizations.
But I am not concerned here to argue the correctness of
those rules. I want only to argue that this format for
rule-making is better than permitting the option of
individualized judicial determinations.

I would apply this same approach to the question of
children's psychiatric hospitalizations. I have written
on this question at some length (see "The Constitution of
the Family," 1979 Supreme Court Review 329); in this
matter, I believe, individualized hearings divert attention
from the needs for (and the propriety of judicial involvement in) fundamental institutional reform in such hospitals.
It seems likely to me that, in practice, judicial commitment hearings supposedly to protect children from parental
"dumping" will tend thoughtlessly to ratify the decisions
of parents and professionals. Such hearings will also
likely intrude on and complicate therapeutic dealings
between the child and the professionals. This intrusion
would not be a persuasive argument against such hearings
if they promised some countervailing benefit to most
children. But I am skeptical of such benefit in most cases.

I mentioned at the outset that the current instinctive
reliance on the lawyerly due process model among some child

advocates is not restricted to parental medical decisions. In closing, let me briefly identify one other area where this model currently holds virtually unquestioned dominance. Consider child custody decisions in divorce cases. Here almost everyone assumes that it is desirable and possible to choose the best possible custodian between father and mother by an individualized inquiry. In contested cases, this inquiry is frequently conducted initially by psychiatrists whose opinions are then reviewed in an adversarial proceeding by a judge. I think we have given insufficient attention to the possibility that, in most cases, the choice between mother and father is incommensurable and that the child's "best interest" simply cannot be known. This possibility would not necessarily argue against individualized hearings; perhaps, like such proceedings for kidney donations, they might be justified as ritual incantations to persuade everyone that the child's interests are being protected even though his parents are destroying his previously intact family.

It seems, however, likely to me that these proceedings are not costless rituals but that they promote and provoke adversarial attitudes among the divorcing spouses that in themselves work against the disputed child's interests. It seems likely that the prospect of such hearings provokes some parents into disputes that they would otherwise settle, however sullenly, if the legal system did not offer them a forum for waging conflict. If we accept the discipline for child custody proceedings that I have proposed earlier, we would set ourselves the task of designing "automatic" custody decisional rules (for example, "the mother always wins" or "under five, the mother wins; over five, the father wins" or "same-sex parent wins"). Each possible rule has problems; each appears to cry out for special exceptions or for precise, psychologically sound individual judgments. But in this context, as in the earlier settings, this appearance may be an illusion -- and not simply a benign illusion, but one that in practice harms many more children than it helps. That, at any rate, is the hypothesis that I would offer for further thought.

Troubling Problems in Medical Ethics: The Third
Volume in a Series on Ethics, Humanism, and Medicine: 109-114
© **1981 Alan R. Liss, Inc., 150 Fifth Ave., New York, NY 10011**

TREATING CHILDREN WITHOUT PARENTAL CONSENT

Arnold S. Relman, M.D.

Editor, New England Journal of Medicine
10 Shattuck Street
Boston, MA

I will say what I have to say as briefly as I can,
hoping thereby to point out as clearly as possible where I
stand and where I may disagree with Professor Burt, so we
can then have more discussion later on.

First of all, it seems to me that a physician's obligation is primarily to help his patient, and not the patient's
parents or next of kin or legal guardian. But in meeting
his obligations to the patient, a physician must consider
the impact of the behavior and attitude of the parents or
next of kin or legal guardian on the patient. The physician
must be particularly aware that young children are essentially
totally dependent on what their parents do, and in weighing
a course of action he must understand that an important part
of the equation is going to be the parent's behavior. Any
recommendation that results in an unhealthy and antagonistic
relationship in the home may be very bad for the child.

The second proposition I suggest is that, except in
emergencies, the physician should serve the patient only with
the patient's consent. Furthermore, I believe that the
consenting patient should be as fully informed as he wishes
to be, but not more than that. Since children cannot give
legal consent, this comment is a bit of a digression. However, I take this opportunity to make what I believe to be
an important point about informed consent. I am opposed to
the notion that the physician ought to tell the patient everything he knows about the patient's condition, regardless of
whether the patient wants to know it all. A good physician
is sensitive to his patient's need for information and he

provides only the information that the patient wants. Trust
in one's physician is therapeutic - it is a very important
part of the therapy in almost every situation. Most patients
understand that, and willingly accept a semi-dependent kind
of relationship with their physician, particularly when they
are very sick. The sicker and more frightened they are, the
more likely they are to want their physician to play a
paternalistic role. But, if the patient does not wish to be
dependent, if the patient wants to know everything there is
to know and wants to participate in decisions, then clearly
it is the physician's obligation to meet the patient's needs.
The good doctor hears what the patient is saying; the patient
may be saying, "Doctor, I trust you, you do what you think
is best for me, and spare me the gory details." Or, the
patient may be saying, "I'm the kind of person who cannot
accept a totally dependent position. I trust you but I do
not want you to withhold anything from me. I want you to
tell me everything." If the patient says that in one way or
another, if he behaves in a way to convey that message to the
doctor, the doctor must be forthright and hold back nothing.
However, physicians should not thrust unwanted information
on their patients. I've seen a great deal of needless pain
inflicted in the name of honesty - doctors believing that
they are doing the right thing by being totally candid and
telling the patient all the brutal facts about his hopeless
disease.

All of the above is an aside. In the present case we
are talking about circumstances where the patient is not
legally competent and the physician must have the consent
of parents or next of kin or legal guardian. When the
patient is an adolescent, the situation is more complicated.
The adolescent patient is old enough to comprehend issues
that a very young child cannot, and to a certain degree is
able to make his own decisions, but he has not yet reached
the age of legal consent. The physician has an obligation
here to gain the consent not only of the parents or legal
guardian, but in a certain sense of the child as well. It
is a very difficult problem to describe in quantitative terms;
at what age do children begin to be able to assume responsibility for dealing with such matters? As Professor Burt
says, some thirteen year olds are very mature, other 13
year olds are not. And some 16 year olds are still immature
children in this sense. So the physician has to make a
judgment, as the child approaches the legal age of consent,
to determine the extent to which the child should participate

in giving consent. And, again, following my principle, the
adolescent child in giving consent should be informed only
to the extent that he wishes to be.

I want to suggest another basic principle. I believe
that competent patients (and to a certain extent the adolescent child would fit my definition of a competent patient)
have a right to decide whether they want treatment or not
and, in a life-threatening situation, whether they want to
have their life artificially prolonged. I believe patients
should be able to walk away from treatment if they don't
want treatment, after they understand fully what they are
doing. As far as children are concerned, though, I don't
believe that parents have the unchallenged right to deny
them life-prolonging or life-saving treatment, even though
parents have that right for themselves.

When parents adamantly refuse treatment that the doctor
believes is necessary for their child, the doctor must weigh
the medical need against the harm that might be done by
pressing ahead with some sort of legal action. Professor
Burt has made clear what that harm can be. It is not just
the harm done by the legal procedure itself, but the harm
done by alienating the parents and making them angry and
resentful; by breaking up the family unity, which may be
essential for the health of the child. The doctor must therefore think very hard about whether the medical situation justifies the step of seeking legal redress. And he should
explore all the non-legal avenues of communication and persuasion that are open to him. A physician confronting parents
who steadfastly refuse to approve treatment he has recommended
for their child must be very sure that the full circumstances
are understood by the parents and that they are fully informed
as to the consequences of their refusal. And he must also
seek other avenues of persuasion; he must talk to other members of the family, to friends, to the minister, or to the
family lawyer. There must be many discussions and a full
exploration of the issues. Furthermore, if the child is an
adolescent he or she must also be involved to the degree
that is appropriate. A few hasty conversations over the
telephone would not meet my definition of full exploration
of the issues. If all this fails, legal action may have to
be taken, but only when clearly needed to protect the child
from serious harm.

I think that I differ with Professor Burt in my definition

of when legal action is needed to protect the child from serious harm. Professor Burt requires, if I understand him correctly, that there be an imminent risk to the child's life, but I would not exclude decisions that would probably jeopardize the quality of the child's later life. Let's say, for example, that the child is presently in reasonably good health but has a congenital heart defect which if not treated now will be crippling later on, and will ultimately shorten his life. Even though there is no immediate threat to the child's health, I would consider that to be an urgent medical situation that might justify legal action. And I also don't agree that the proposed medical intervention must be a certain cure. Very few medical interventions are. Medicine is essentially a probabilistic art, and we have to be satisfied most of the time with doing things that we think are probably going to help. Professor Burt would also require that the side effects be minimal. Well, lots of useful treatments have more than minimal side effects, and here again I think that Professor Burt's criteria may be a bit too stringent. If the weight of medical opinion supports the treatment as being clearly in the child's best interest, if the great majority of competent physicians presented with the case would say that the child should be treated in a certain way, then I think there is reason to take some action if the parents refuse.

Now, what about the case under discussion here? The child is an adolescent, 14 years old, and therefore should be involved in giving his informed consent. I believe that Dr. Springer should have talked at length and in person with the boy. A brief conversation over the phone is not enough. Furthermore, it's not clear that the parents were fully informed either. It is not clear to me from the case history whether the parents were refusing because they thought they knew a better way to treat their son, or because they thought that no helpful medical treatment was available and they wanted him to be allowed to die in peace. It is not clear from the protocol what the parents thought or whether they really fully understood the situation. Did they really know that there is not a shred of evidence that any diet or natural food or vitamins would influence the course of their son's leukemia? Dr. Springer had an obligation to explain all this to the parents and to be sure that they understood what medical treatment had to offer. He had an obligation to know exactly why they were refusing his advice.

The trouble with this case, and I assume that the facts were chosen expressly for this reason, is that it is in the borderline zone for medical treatment of leukemia. The boy was 14 years old and we know that the older a child is, the less favorable is the prognosis for acute lymphoblastic leukemia; older children respond less well to treatment than younger children. Also, he had T-cell lymphoblastic leukemia and we know that this form of acute leukemia does not have as good a prognosis as other kinds of lymphoblastic leukemia. Furthermore, he had already been on treatment for 16 months and was in remission. The optimal therapy is thought to be about three years of maintenance therapy after induction of remission, but there really aren't any good data to say that the boy would be worse off stopping at 16 months than at 30 months, or at three years. So the medical situation here is a little fuzzy.

What would I do in this particular case? I think I would have done a lot more than Dr. Springer did in talking with the parents. He conferred with them by phone, but I would have confronted them personally. I also would have talked to the patient, I would have involved other people in the discussion and I would have explored with the boy and with the parents what they thought was so bad about the side effects. The fact of the matter is that most of the side effects of chemotherapy are tolerable and they can be kept under reasonable control by appropriate medical management.

Often what lies behind such a strong negative reaction by the parents is not concern with the effects of chemo-therapy, but something else - some more irrational and emo-tional objection. It might have been helpful to explore with the parents why they were really objecting. Was the boy himself really objecting that much to chemotherapy? It is interesting that the mother said that <u>she</u> had nightmares about bringing the child to the clinic. Did the boy have nightmares, or did he sleep quite peacefully? The important question here is not the mother's state of mind but the boy's.

So I respond this way: The medical evidence in this case is not quite clear enough to warrant going to court to ask that the judge hand down an order telling the parents that they must allow the doctors to treat this boy; but there is no question in my mind that most physicians experi-enced in the treatment of leukemia would feel uncomfortable stopping treatment after 16 months. If he were my son, I certainly would want him treated for at least 30 months. Therefore, I would feel an obligation to persuade the parents to go along.

But if the parents refused, whether I would push it to the point of a court order would have to depend on the details of the case. One would need to get the sense of what was going on in that family: What kind of a family is it? What would be the consequences of going to court? Would such action in this case have all the bad effects that Professor Burt discussed (in which case I might back away), or on balance would going to court be better?

In conclusion, I would say that I do not fear court proceedings as much as Professor Burt does in cases such as this. However, I stand squarely on his side in most circumstances, agreeing with him that most of the time the courts are not able to deal with complicated medical decisions. Too often they make matters worse, no matter what they decide. In this kind of case, though, I think there is a place for the courts. When the doctors recommend treatment and the parents refuse, there may be reason to go to court because parents do not have the right to inflict the medical consequences of their irrational biases on their children. I'm not saying that it is always irrational to refuse to follow your doctor's recommendations - not at all. What I am saying, however, is that if he is able to understand the implications an adolescent ought to have the right to make up his own mind about whether he wishes to follow the doctor's advice. A minor's right to the benefits of medical treatment - if the benefits are clear and important to his health - should not be denied him by his parents. To condemn a child to ill-health, or possibly even to death, simply because his parents have some kind of emotional problem seems to me unjust. So I am willing to take certain risks with the use of the court process that perhaps Professor Burt is not.

**Troubling Problems in Medical Ethics: The Third
Volume in a Series on Ethics, Humanism, and Medicine: 115–116
© 1981 Alan R. Liss, Inc., 150 Fifth Ave., New York, NY 10011**

DISCUSSION SUMMARY: TREATING CHILDREN WITHOUT PARENTAL CONSENT

Rachel Lipson
Program Director, CEHM
University of Michigan
Ann Arbor, Michigan

Most groups felt that the doctor should not go to
court to force treatment on Bobby. One group member who
expressed the opinion of most of the participants said,
"Bobby seems to agree with his parents, and if he doesn't
want treatment then Dr. Springer has no right to force it on
him." However, one physician contended that fourteen year
olds are not really capable of abstract thinking, and are
thus not capable of making important decisions about their
own medical care.

The one group that supported Dr. Springer's lawsuit
agreed with Dr. Relman that it is difficult to tell from
the case why the parents were refusing treatment and whether
Bobby really agreed with them. Members of this group believed
that until the physician had had a chance to talk with both
Bobby and his parents, in person, he should not allow the
Smiths' decision to stand. If, after using all other
available means, the doctor still was not convinced by the
Smiths then they felt he should go to court. One student in
this group said, "It just isn't fair for a fourteen year
old to die because he and his parents don't quite understand
what is going on medically."

Although several groups discussed the dangers of going
to court to which Professor Burt alluded, none seemed to
resolve this issue. One group did, however, feel that the
development of rules for such situations would be even more
dangerous than case-by-case adversarial proceedings, because
each family is special and deserves special attention. One
group secretary also noted that all the lawyers in his group

had voted to go to court and did not seem to fear the system to be as biased as Burt claimed.

Other issues that were discussed in several groups included: paternalism, what should have been done if Bobby were four or twenty-four, rather than fourteen, and whether the case would have been any different if Mrs. Smith had been a physician. Some groups were concerned that the physician would always act in a paternalistic manner, even if the Smiths had valid reasons for refusing therapy, that "doctors feel that they somehow know what is best and they don't listen to anyone else." One group, which discussed what should have been done if Bobby were four or twenty-four, all felt that the doctor should clearly have gone to court if the boy were four, while if he were twenty-four, Bobby could have made his own decisions and the doctor would have had no right to interfere. Most group members also agreed that even if Mrs. Smith were a physician she would still have been unable to be objective about this case because of her maternal feelings for Bobby.

Troubling Problems in Medical Ethics: The Third
Volume in a Series on Ethics, Humanism, and Medicine: 117–118
© **1981 Alan R. Liss, Inc., 150 Fifth Ave., New York, NY 10011**

INTRODUCTION: THE DECISION TO RESUSCITATE - SLOWLY

Marc D. Basson
Director, CEHM
University of Michigan
Ann Arbor, Michigan

The "slow code" is a medical practice almost unknown
outside medical circles. Punning on the "code/no code"
decision which sums up the appropriateness of resuscitative
efforts for a given patient, the slow code is applied to
patients whose prognosis makes them unsuitable for resuscitation in the doctor's view while other factors necessitate
at least the semblance of a resuscitative attempt. In the
case presented for discussion here, for instance, a terminally
ill young woman has therapeutic support withdrawn, undergoes
cardiopulmonary arrest, and then dies while the "code team"
moves with deliberate slowness.

This case is particularly agonizing because the patient
remains conscious until the arrest, but a slow code is never
an easy thing. Deliberate here means not only intentional
but also carefully considered. It is the physician's un-
raveling of a Gordian knot tying together a hopeless prognosis
with a family's apparently irrational desire that life be
prolonged at all costs. Either the family has refused to
approve "do not resuscitate" status for the patient or the
doctor believes they would refuse if asked. Yet the physician
knows that the situation is hopeless, that the patient is
either unconscious or uncomfortable, and that thousands of
dollars of hospital costs accumulate each day. The slow
code is an attempt to cut the knot, pretending to the family
that "we did all we could" while allowing the patient to
die.

For Martin Benjamin, a philosopher from Michigan State
University with extensive hospital experience, the essence

of the slow code is paternalism. It takes decision-making power away from patients, family or designated proxy. Benjamin believes and argues strongly that the patient must have the right to choose his fate, even if his choice is only to abide by his doctor's advice. Benjamin rejects considerations of scarce medical resources and cost-effectiveness as irrelevant to choices within an individual doctor-patient relationship. He also argues that the slow code is essentially deceitful and that this too militates against its practice.

David Dantzker disagrees. An astute clinician with a long interest in intensive care medicine, he begins by trying to give his audience a feeling for the realities of the situation from the physician's perspective. Informed consent is almost impossible to obtain from an intubated patient in an intensive care unit, Dantzker claims. (Benjamin disagrees.) In addition, Dantzker suggests that we may be attributing too much significance to the decision to carry out a slow code, for the patient will certainly die soon regardless of our intervention. Ultimately, however, Dantzker accepts Benjamin's characterization of the slow code and refuses to let it dissuade him. "If these arguments sound paternalistic," Dantzker writes, "I offer no excuses since medicine is by its nature a paternalistic profession." Resuscitation is not as simple as code/no code, Dantzker points out. Rather, the question of how hard or long to work on a dying patient is a complicated one, necessarily decided by the physician at the bedside. Given the complexity of the decision, Dantzker argues that only the doctor is competent to choose in cases such as the one described.

**Troubling Problems in Medical Ethics: The Third
Volume in a Series on Ethics, Humanism, and Medicine: 119–122
© 1981 Alan R. Liss, Inc., 150 Fifth Ave., New York, NY 10011**

THE DECISION TO RESUSCITATE - SLOWLY

CASE FOR DISCUSSION

8/24/80: Senior Resident Admit Note (excerpt)
     Joanne Sterling is a 33 year old white female police-
woman struck by a car at approximately 2:00 p.m. today while
directing traffic. She sustained multiple injuries and
required cardiopulmonary resuscitation and epinephrine in
the ambulance. On arrival she was found to have bilateral
pneumothoraces, flail chest with multiple rib fractures.
Open fractures of the left hip and right humerus were also
noted. She was stabilized in the Emergency Room with intubation and ventilation, bilateral chest tubes, 2 units of
type specific blood and 10 units of cross-matched blood.
Other diagnostic studies were normal and she was transferred
to Surgical ICU for monitoring and treatment.

8/29/80: Pulmonary Resident Transfer Note (excerpt)
     Vital signs remained unstable in the SICU and the
patient's temperature spiked to 102°. Blood and sputum
cultures grew pseudomonas. She is being transferred to the
Respiratory ICU for treatment of her massive pulmonary
infection and for weaning from the ventilator (so far unsuccessful).

9/5/80: Resident Progress Note
     Mrs. Sterling's maximal temperature today was 103.5° on
a cooling blanket. Latest blood cultures are growing pseudomonas, serratia, and candida. Will switch antibiotics to
gentamicin, carbenicillin, amphotericin in an effort to
control her infection. Prognosis guarded.

9/12/80: Student Progress Note
     Pulmonary function continues to deteriorate, now requir-
ing maximal ventilatory support (IMV16, FIO_2 90%, PEEP 15).
Pt. seems to be developing respiratory distress syndrome, a
condition characterized by progressive stiffening of the
lungs and secondary inability to inhale enough oxygen, all
related to the trauma suffered during the accident. Prognosis
is poor.

9/18/80:
     Left chest tube placed for pneumothorax secondary to
use of maximal ventilator.

10/1/80: Cross Cover Note, 2 a.m.
     Pt. became confused and disconnected herself from the
ventilator for approximately 3 minutes. Arterial oxygenation
in specimen drawn just after reconnection incompatible with
life. Fortunately, later gases on ventilator were better.
Neurological exam one hour later, however, was entirely
normal. Patient was alert, oriented, and communicated
appropriately by pointing to letters on a large alphabet
board and thus spelling out her words.

10/25/80: Intern Off Service Note (excerpt)
     Her original trauma-related problems have almost completely
resolved. However, her lungs are so stiff from respiratory
distress syndrome that it is impossible for her to breathe
on her own. Her on-going infection is being controlled with
triple antibiotics but we are making no progress in curing
it. The prognosis is therefore grim and the ethical dilemma
of how aggressive to be in her management still remains. I
am told that her hospital stay has already cost over $50,000!!
The present policy is to continue aggressive treatment and
support as her mental status is still good. She is alert
and communicates appropriately, if awkwardly, by letter
board. She is presently considered competent to sign her
own consent. Her husband comes in once a week with her
eight year old daughter and seems quite concerned that
everything possible be done. He has been told of the prognosis.
Good luck with this interesting and most troubling patient.

10/28/80: Psychiatry Consult
     Called to see patient after she reportedly became con-
fused and attempted to extubate herself. She seems coherent
and appropriate at the present time and does not recall the
incident. We were able to "talk" for two hours this afternoon

by means of her letter board and she expressed her anxiety
over death. She notes that her staff rarely talks with her
anymore and wonders if this is because they think she will
die soon. (Has she been told her prognosis?)

The picture of ICU psychosis is one of intermittent
disorientation and confusion related to lack of defined
contact with her environment. The best treatment is attention.
Allow her to ventilate mentally as well as physically. Talk
to her whenever possible. Keep a radio playing in her room
on a station that gives the news and time frequently. Keep
a calendar in plain sight.

11/6/80: Senior Staff Note
After over two months in the RICU, it has become obvious
that Mrs. Sterling's pulmonary fibrosis is severe, irreversible,
and incompatible with life. Even with maximal ventilatory
support, her continued disseminated infection makes her
death within a few months a virtual certainty. Thus, our
current aggressive therapy seems neither rational nor cost-
effective.

Therefore, after extensive discussions among the ward
team and nursing staff caring for the patient, we have decided
to discontinue antibiotics, intravenous fluids, and further
blood testing. This decision has not been discussed with
either the patient or her family as in my judgment this
would be needless cruelty, especially given the patient's
constant anxiety over dying and the guilt which might accrue
to the husband who agreed to let her die. We have no choice,
for the therapy cannot go on forever and others are waiting
for the ICU beds. However, patient remains on full code
status (i.e., full resuscitation) for legal reasons as she
has not given consent for No Code.

11/8/80: ICU Intern Death Note (excerpt)
Patient arrested at 6:03 p.m. after apparently accidental
self-extubation while her restraints were off and her bed
was being cleaned. Resuscitation team was notified and
arrived at 6:05. I advised the team of Mrs. Sterling's prognosis and we then decided to comply with the legal requirements of resuscitation for this full code status patient but
without undue haste, given her condition. The patient was
intubated at 6:15 and resuscitation commenced. It was noted
that the EKG monitor failed to show a heartbeat at 6:17;
this was confirmed with a standard EEG machine and closed

chest cardiac massage was then started at 6:21. The patient
was pronounced dead at 6:30 after resuscitation had failed.

"Codes" or cardiopulmonary resuscitation attempts may
be routinely prolonged for over thirty minutes with favorable
results. The patient is typically intubated within one or
two minutes by the most competent person present. Was it
appropriate for the patient's resuscitation to be slowed and
abbreviated because of her other medical problems? Should
the patient or her family have been consulted about the
decision to discontinue therapy or about possible options
should the patient's condition worsen acutely? Should they
have been informed of the decisions being made even if not
allowed to choose? Would it make a difference if the patient's
life expectancy with adequate support therapy were a matter
of hours rather than months? What if it were a matter of
years with adequate ventilation support and antibiotics?
What role does the scarcity of ICU beds and health care play
in your assessment? Is it important that the patient suffered
her initial accident while working as a policewoman and
serving society?

(Case prepared by Marc Basson.)

Troubling Problems in Medical Ethics: The Third
Volume in a Series on Ethics, Humanism, and Medicine: 123–129
© 1981 Alan R. Liss, Inc., 150 Fifth Ave., New York, NY 10011

PATIENT AUTONOMY AND THE DECISION TO RESUSCITATE "WITHOUT
UNDUE HASTE"

Martin Benjamin, Ph.D.

Department of Philosophy

Michigan State University, East Lansing

This case bristles with ethical issues and we could
spend many profitable sessions examing them. Since time is
limited, however, I will focus on three different, but related, questions that are central to any sustained inquiry
into the case.

The three questions are: (1) To what extent should the
patient and her family be involved in the decision not to
resuscitate? (2) Were the decisions made by the staff on
November 6 and 8 justifiable? and (3) At what level, if
any, and for what reasons, if any, should economic considerations, including the high cost of Mrs. Sterling's care
and the scarcity of ICU beds, play a role in the decision?

WHOSE DECISION?

It would be a mistake to turn too quickly to the fate-
ful decisions confronting the staff on November 6 and 8.
For this would presuppose that there is nothing questionable
about the way Mrs. Sterling was treated until then. But, as
I will suggest, the agonizing decisions of November 6 and 8
may have been unnecessary if the patient and her family had
been included in the decision-making during the preceding
months.

As is becoming more widely recognized, competent adult
patients have a right to accept or refuse medical treatment,
even life-saving or life-prolonging treatment (Veatch, 1976).
This is a right originating in common law rules relating to

battery and based philosophically on the principle of autonomy and the right to self-determination. Although not all
patients are able and willing to exercise this right, many
are able and willing to make such decisions even within the
context of intensive care (Imbus and Zawacki, 1976; Rabkin,
et. al., 1976). Nonetheless, extreme caution should be exercised to ensure that decisions to terminate treatment in
this context are fully informed and genuinely autonomous
(Jackson and Youngner, 1979). Thus it is important that
physicians be willing to undertake a "time consuming and potentially painful dialogue" with the patient and his or her
family (Jackson and Youngner, 1980).

In the case before us we are provided with no evidence
to suggest that Mrs. Sterling was not competent to decide
whether, all things considered, the possible benefits of
continued treatment were, to her, worth the burdens and
costs. Moreover, entries into her chart on October 1, 25,
and 28 strongly suggest that she was competent to make such
a decision. Why, therefore, was she apparently left out of
the decision-making? Assuming that she was competent, the
question of continued treatment should have begun to be
carefully and tactfully broached no later than September 12
when it was noted in the chart that "Prognosis is poor."

Although there are possible considerations that may
have justified bypassing Mrs. Sterling's right to accept or
refuse further treatment, my reading of the case does not
reveal any of them. It is not, for example, sufficient to
appeal at this stage to "the patient's constant anxiety
over dying and the guilt that might accrue to the husband
who agreed to let her die" that was noted in the chart on
November 6 when the decision was made to stop antibiotic
treatment. For if we take rights seriously, as I believe we
should, the fact that someone would be saddened and dis-
tressed by information to which he or she has a right is
not sufficient reason to withhold it. Sadness, distress,
anxiety, and possible guilt on the part of the husband are
natural responses to situations of this kind. But they are
emotions to be acknowledged and worked through by the patient, family, and staff and not to be avoided at any cost.

Moreover, it may well be that Mrs. Sterling's anxiety
was in part aggravated by the failure of the staff to discuss, supportively but candidly, her prognosis with her. As

the psychiatric consultation of October 28 suggests, Mrs. Sterling was not allowed to discuss in words what was conveyed by the behavior of the staff--viz., that she was dying. Moreover, it is possible that the three occasions on which she disconnected herself from the respirator were also attempts to convey in action what was believed to be forbidden to express in words. A failure then, as the psychiatrist put it, "to allow her to ventilate mentally as well as physically" may have contributed to her anxiety.

It is important to note, in this regard, that the extent to which a patient can exercise autonomy in the medical setting is, in part, a function of the support and encouragement of the staff. Just as teachers who supportively expect their students to do well always seem to have "better students" than those who expect them to do poorly, so too it is likely that the extent to which patients will be able to make well-informed and genuinely autonomous decisions to accept or refuse medical care will be a function of the expectations and support of the staff. Thus, it is not unreasonable to assume that Mrs. Sterling's passivity was in part a product of the way she was treated.

Of course, the press of affairs in an ICU and the awkwardness of communicating by letter board make the sort of dialogue I am suggesting especially difficult. But entries in the chart for October 1, 25, and 28 imply that it would have been possible.

Finally, let me make clear that I am not suggesting that the patient had an obligation to be candidly informed of her prognosis and an obligation to decide to accept or refuse treatment, but only that she had rights to them. She may, if she wishes, decide to waive these rights. But she cannot do this without being given the opportunity to do so. And, as far as I can tell, she was not given this opportunity.

THE STAFF'S DECISION

Let us now suppose that, having been fully and supportively informed of their rights, both Mrs. Sterling and her husband have elected to waive them. They have made it clear that they want the staff to do whatever they think is

best and they do not want to be troubled by medical information or agonizing decisions. Although I am not favorably
disposed to such situations and hope their numbers will diminish in the future, they can occur. Supposing this to be
the case, then, what can we say about the decisions made by
the staff on November 6 and 8?

The first of these was to discontinue antibiotics, intravenous fluids, and further blood testing and the second
was to respond to the legal requirements for a full code
"without undue haste." Underlying each of these decisions
was the belief that there was little reason to continue Mrs.
Sterling's treatment longer than was legally necessary.
Not only was she suffering but further treatment, given her
condition, seemed pointlessly expensive and prevented others, who would receive greater medical benefit, from occu-
pying her place in ICU.

At this stage, given our supposition that the patient
and her husband have fully transferred their right to make
decisions to the staff, there is no need to discuss the decisions with them. The author of the senior staff note of
November 6 is probably correct to note that at this point
this would be "needless cruelty."

As for the decisions themselves, the first thing to
note is that they both involve negative acts aimed at
shortening life. This is not, however, to say that they
are morally wrong, but rather to stress that Mrs. Sterling's
death, in this case, is no less attributable to human agency than if she were given a lethal injection. Although
limitations of space do not allow the development of the
relevant arguments, the bare difference between a positive
act, such as giving a lethal injection, and a negative act,
such as deliberately withholding life-prolonging treatment,
is not relevant from a moral point of view (Rachels, 1975;
Benjamin, 1979). Thus, legal considerations aside, deliberately allowing Mrs. Sterling to die in these circumstances
is no more justified than ending her life with a lethal injection; and ending her life with a lethal injection is no
worse, from a moral point of view, than deciding to respond
to her arrest "without undue haste." I mention this not so
much to decide the moral issue, but rather to emphasize the
momentousness of the "decision to resuscitate--slowly." For
we deceive ourselves if we believe that allowing someone to
die requires less in the way of moral justification on the

part of physicians than actively hastening death.

Secondly, the decision to respond to Mrs. Sterling's arrest "without undue haste" is tainted by the fact that it required dissembling (This aspect of the case was brought to my attention by Robert J. Levine, M.D.). The resuscitation team and the ICU intern who wrote the death note performed a sham code. Sissela Bok has forcefully argued that each deceptive act, no matter how apparently innocuous, has a corrosive effect on the sort of trust that is necessary for the preservation of essential, but fragile, social bonds; and thus each such act bears a heavy burden of justification (Bok, 1978). Why then, we may ask, was it necessary in this case to conduct a resuscitative charade? If allowing Mrs. Sterling to die was justifiable, why try to hide it? If the legal or institutional rules require dissembling in order to do what is morally right, why not challenge them openly and directly? For to rely on pretense suggests that one believes that what one is doing is wrong. Moreover, even if the ends of one's (positive or negative) action are not in themselves wrong, acting deceptively is, unless justified, wrong in itself.

ECONOMIC CONSIDERATIONS

I will assume that the high cost of specialized medical care and the question of the just and efficient utilization of ICU beds is, and will remain, an important problem in health care. Certainly the entries into the chart on October 25 and November 7 suggest that economic considerations may have played a role in Mrs. Sterling's case. But although I agree that such considerations cannot be ignored, I have some reservations about physicians taking it upon themselves, in an ad hoc and unregulated fashion, to make judgements about the allocation of funds and resources which are best made at a different level of the health care system.

Following Charles Fried, I think it is important to distinguish three levels in the health care system: (1) the providers of primary care; (2) the hospital or clinic administrator; and (3) the government official (Fried, 1974). Questions of allocation, Fried argues, should be made at levels (2) and (3) to assure that distributions will be equitable and efficient and to avoid undermining the trust

and personal loyalty that are essential to the doctor-patient
relationship at level (1). The patient should be justified
in believing that his or her physician is doing everything
within his or her power to respond to the patient's informed, legitimate requests for care. And where matters of social equity or efficiency in the allocation of scarce resources lead to policy decisions at levels (2) and (3) that
limit the doctor's efforts, his or her personal fidelity to
the patient is thus uncompromised. To give physicians at
level (1) the responsibility for making such decisions,
Fried suggests, will not only undermine overall equity and
efficiency, but it will also strain the vital bond between
doctor and patient.

Moreover, to leave such decisions entirely to the
discretion of individual physicians is also likely to
lead to decisions that are arbitrary or (unintentionally)
biased. One cannot, for example, overlook the fact that
studies have shown that social factors such as age, class,
appearance, sobriety, etc., are often correlated with the
degree of vigor with which patients are resuscitated in
emergency rooms (Sudnow, 1960; Simpson, 1976). And even
the most conscientious, fair-minded physician will find it
difficult at the personal level to expunge all of the effects of transference, positive and negative, from such
decisions.

Therefore, although economic considerations may become factors in cases of this kind, they should, I believe,
be addressed mainly as matters of policy at the appropriate
levels and with the appropriate systematic concern for efficiency and impartiality rather than at the bedside. As
for this case, however, my hunch is that if, from the very
beginning, the patient had been placed squarely in the center of decision-making and given appropriate staff support,
the economic question may never have arisen.

REFERENCES

Benjamin M (1979). Moral agency and negative acts in
    medicine. In Pritchard M, Robison W (eds): "Medical Re-
    sponsibility," Clifton, NJ: Humana Press, pp. 169-80.
Bok S (1978). "Lying: Moral Choice in Public and Private
    Life." New York: Pantheon, passim.

Fried C (1974). "Medical Experimentation." Amsterdam: North-Holland, pp. 116-32.

Imbus S, Zawacki B (1977). Autonomy for burned patients when survival is unprecedented. N.E.J.M 297:308-11.

Jackson DL, Youngner S (1979). Patient autonomy and "death with dignity," N.E.J.M 301:404-408.

Jackson DL, Youngner S (1980). Family wishes and patient autonomy. Hastings Center Report 10:21-22.

Rabkin MT, Gillerman G, Rice NR (1976). Orders not to resuscitate. N.E.J.M 295:364-66.

Rachels J (1975). Active and passive euthanasia. N.E.J.M 292:78-80.

Simpson MA (1976). Brought in dead. Omega 7:243-48.

Sudnow D (1967). "Passing On: The Social Organization of Dying." Englewood Cliffs, NJ: Prentice-Hall, pp. 98-102

Veatch RM (1976). "Death, Dying, and the Biological Revolution." New Haven: Yale, pp. 116-63.

**Troubling Problems in Medical Ethics: The Third
Volume in a Series on Ethics, Humanism, and Medicine: 131-140
© 1981 Alan R. Liss, Inc., 150 Fifth Ave., New York, NY 10011**

THE DECISION TO RESUSCITATE - SLOWLY

David R. Dantzker, M.D.
Assistant Professor of Internal Medicine
University of Michigan

Ann Arbor, Michigan

When first asked to discuss this case, I must say that
I was somewhat hesitant. However, I finally accepted the
challenge because I thought it would be interesting to try to
formalize my thinking on a subject which I deal with intimately
every day, but prior to this only on an empirical basis.

Decision making in medicine has for a long time been the
special province of the physician, and recent intrusions into
that domain by philosophers, lawyers and judges have led to
reactions from the medical community which have ranged all
the way from fear to anger. People asking questions such as
how long should we allow doctors at the bedside to decide
life and death issues are both provocative and difficult for
the physician to consider unemotionally. And yet questions
regarding the role of the patient, the role of the family,
and even the role of the community and the courts in medical
decision making are legitimate concerns and have been long
overdue.

While we will be talking today about the broad question
of decision making in the critically ill patient I see as my
charge to bring up a very specific question related to this
case, and one that I think Marc Basson had in mind when he
chose it. That question is whether or not it is ever justified for a physician to make decisions concerning the appropriateness of resuscitation on his own without consulting
the patient or family. Further, if the physician is ever so
justified, is the use of what we call a "qualified resuscitative attempt" or in the parlance of the hospital, a "slow
code", ever an appropriate vehicle for carrying out this
decision?

Since the goal of this portion of the session is to provide a framework for further discussion, I will try to provide some insight into one clinician's view of this problem, and raise what I hope will be a few provocative questions. Because the case is somewhat complicated, I thought I would begin by reviewing the case history and explain to you some of the terminology so that we will all be starting from the same point of reference.

This patient was involved in an auto accident and sustained multiple, severe, traumatic injuries. These resulted in extensive fractures of the bones of both of her legs and her right arm. She had multiple broken ribs and had also suffered contusions (bruises) to both lungs resulting in what we call bilateral pneumothoracies, or holes in both sides of her lungs. Because of this, the air she was breathing was pouring into her chest cavity. It is also likely that she suffered trauma to her heart, as we are told in the protocol that she suffered a cardiac arrest at the scene and was resuscitated prior to being brought to the hospital. When she reached the hospital, she was placed in traction - by this I mean both legs and arms were stabilized by the use of pins through the bones and various kinds of weights and pulleys. She was also placed on mechanical ventilation because the damage to her lungs made her unable to breath on her own. The remaining hospital course while quite complicated can be summarized fairly simply. The patient spent two and a half months in an intensive care unit during which time she had multiple episodes of pneumonia, sepsis (by which I mean systemic bacterial infection in her blood stream) pulmonary edema (fluid in her lungs) and persistent hypoxemia (the oxygen tension in her blood remained low despite efforts by physicians, both with mechanical ventilation and by increasing the amount of oxygen, to bring this level of oxygen in the blood up to reasonable amounts). In addition, she had the persistent holes in her lungs which failed to heal. These holes required tubes to be placed and required special forms of mechanical ventilation in order to provide enough air in and out of her lungs to maintain adequate oxygenation. Because of all of these problems, in particular the episodes of pneumonia and pulmonary edema and the very high levels of oxygen that were necessary to keep her alive, she developed what we call "severe pulmonary fibrosis". In other words, her lungs, instead of being soft and balloon-like, became scarred and very stiff. It was difficult to inflate them, even using the very high pressures that the

mechanical ventilator could generate. In fact, a special
ventilator was necessary to develop the kinds of pressures
that were necessary to move sufficient air into her lungs to
keep her alive. During the period of her hospitalization,
she was intermittently confused and disoriented, and it was
the impression of the physicians and nurses that she rarely
understood what was said to her. A number of times she
removed her endotracheal tube with her one free hand or disconnected herself from the mechanical ventilator.

Her husband found this situation very difficult to deal
with. In the beginning he visited reasonably often, but as
time wore on, his visits decreased in frequency and he found
it more difficult to go into the room. His time in the room
became much shorter and his ability to discuss his wife's
medical situation with physicians deteriorated. In the end
he was showing up for very short periods of time, at very
odd hours of the day, and he was very difficult to reach by
phone.

About 2-1/2 months into her hospital course, after much
discussion, it was agreed by the attending medical staff, the
consulting physicians who had been following her, and the
nurses in the intensive care unit, that the severe pulmonary
fibrosis was irreversible. She would never be able to exist
off of this very special ventilator, and in a short time,
one of the multiple episodes of sepsis, pulmonary edema or
pneumonia would prove fatal. Her blood pressure had been
falling slowly and her hypoxemia was gradually getting worse.
A decision was made that the patient was not a candidate for
resuscitation in the event of another cardiac arrest. It
was also decided not to confront the patient or her husband
with the decision, a factor which provides the basis for our
decision. Because of this decision, conservative management
was provided; which in this case meant that sedation was
provided; analgesia was continued and maintenance interven-
ous fluids were given to maintain a normal state of hydration.
However, no antibiotics or extraordinary means of cardiac
resuscitation were to be employed. Soon after this the
patient suffered a cardiac arrest following another episode
of extubation. While the apparent slow motion of the resuscitative effort has been a little bit fictionalized for its
dramatic effects, a decision had definitely been made before
this happened to be less than vigorous in the event of an
arrest.

We live in a time when it is common to attempt the promulgation of laws and rules to govern every imaginable human endeavor. For that reason I will use as a framework for my discussion a group of standards that were proposed by Rabkin, et al (Rabkin, Gillerman, Rice 1978) to regulate decisions concerning "no Code" orders.

Since the physician's traditional duty is to preserve life, it is appropriate at the onset to ask the question whether or not a decision not to resuscitate is ever a defensible one. Robert Veatch in his book DEATH, DYING AND THE BIOLOGICAL REVOLUTION (Veatch, 1976) asked the question whether it is still morally acceptable to die in this technological age. However, there are now few enlightened people who would argue that technology must always be applied to its maximal limit to prolong the life of each and every patient. This is especially true now when fewer and fewer people die outside of hospitals. If one looks at the statistics, we find that over the last 20 or 30 years, less and less people actually are allowed to die at home. More than 60% of the patients dying in this country, now die at some medical institution, whether it be a hospital or a nursing home. (Lerner 1970)

Traditional ethical teachings allow that administration of heroic and extraordinary means to preserve the life of the terminally ill is not necessary and under certain circumstances one is even permitted to remove temporary hindrances to death. If you go back in Western ethical tradition, this is spoken of time and again. In this case, we have a patient who was terminally ill. She was clearly dying at the time the decision not to resuscitate was made. Her lungs had been damaged beyond all hopes of healing, and it was only a matter of time before she became infected with some resistant organism or fell victim to one of the other catastrophes that abound in the modern day intensive care unit. This patient, I think we should realize, is not a Karen Quinlan. She is not a vegetative but otherwise stable patient in whom the question is whether or not to withdraw life support. This is a patient who sits on the knife-edge of survival awaiting only that final push that will lead to her death.

Given the premise that it is ethical, on occasion, to withhold extraordinary care we may ask who should decide whether or not death is so inevitable that resuscitative attempts or efforts may no longer be warranted?

Sometimes the patient can initiate this decision. The patient's right to refuse treatment is a well-recognized right as part of his/her right of privacy. The courts in this country have always recognized the fact that with the exception of some extenuating circumstances, for example, when a third party's welfare is also involved, the patient has the right to determine when he/she no longer wishes to be treated. I think that the medical community has the necessity to respect that right. Occasionally, however, the situation arises (as I feel it did in this case) that the patient is unable to make rational decisions or to communicate their feelings either because of an altered state of consciousness or abnormal mental function. When this happens, the burden of decision falls, by necessity, to the physician. This is appropriate, since diagnosing illness and determining prognosis and treatment are what the physician is trained for and what the patient is paying the doctor to do. There is no way that the doctor should be relieved of this responsibility. The establishment of the doctor/patient relationship, no matter how informed or how intelligent the patient, is based upon a trust that the physician will recommend and do what he thinks is in the best interest of the patient. Rabkin, in his article on resuscitation (Rabkin, Gillerman, Rice, 1976) suggests that it is possible for the physician to relieve himself of part of this burden of decision-making by asking the approval of a committee. This committee of medical professionals made up of physicians and nurses would look at the data and then decide whether the decision not to resuscitate is correct. However, does such a committee really improve the decision-making ability or relieve the doctor of any moral burden? What is the data base that this committee uses to make their decisions? By and large the data base is the physician who brings the question to the committee. I think that it is unlikely, especially in small hospitals, where the medical community is very close, that a committee of this sort is going to take a position opposite from the doctor who brings the case to it. In addition, I'm not certain that there is any a priori reason to believe that discussion by this type of committee would result in a more appropriate decision than that made by the patient's physician alone. This is especially true because the physician has at least had direct contact with the patient, and hopefully has made his decision on both medical and moral grounds.

This question of having physicians make moral decisions
seems to be a real bugaboo in the death and dying literature.
People seem to feel that physicians are certainly able to
make medical decisions, but they shouldn't make any moral
decisions. For some reason some wish to exclude doctors
from the moral process. I would quote Dr. Arnold Relman
from a recent article that he wrote in the American Journal
of Law and Medicine (Relman 1979) in which he said that
"The moral and technical aspects of medical practice are
frequently inseparable for the simple reason that people are
not machines. Few important clinical decisions can be made
properly without consideration of the humanity of the
patient, and this inevitably requires the weighing of moral
issues. A purely technical physician could be a menace
because his judgement would lack compassion and human
understanding. I doubt that many patients would feel comfortable with such a person. They expect more than a technical service when they consult their physician."

Another suggestion has been made by Allen Buchanan in
the same issue of the American Journal of Law and Medicine
(Buchanan 1979) to carry this committee idea even further.
He feels that such a committee should include not only
physicians, but psychiatrists, psychologists, lawyers, lay
people, moral philosophers, people who have had to make
this decision before, etc. In addition, he felt that not
only should they help make this decision but some people
should be required to take an adversary role in the proceeding. I can't see that this would be a workable solution to
a problem that in one way or another comes up frequently in
the general hospital. It has never been shown that committee decisions come out better than a decision made by a
single dedicated, well trained physician.

To carry this question of making the decision not to
resuscitate just a bit further, we could ask whether or not
the decision is really that important. That may sound
strange since we are talking about problems of life and
death, but is the decision to resuscitate or not really
crucial? In the case we are discussing today, we could ask,
did the decision to resuscitate slowly or not at all
actually change the inevitable outcome for this patient?
Are the arguments about code or no code really an exercise
in self delusion; in believing that we can make these kinds
of decisions and that they really make a difference. Do
we actually have the ability, despite all the sophisticated

equipment, drugs, and techniques, to really influence life
and death decisions at this point in a patient's life. I
would suggest that in fact most often we don't. If we
eliminate patients who have simple cardiac arrests due to
electrical malfunctions of their hearts (for example ventri-
cular fibrillation due to myocardial infarction) and instead
look at patients with problems like our patient today, we
will find that most of these patients will not survive a
resuscitative attempt, no matter how much we do or how
well we do it. Even the patients in whom we are able to
reestablish a normal or functional heart rhythm, most will
never leave the hospital. Far and away the majority of
those patients will die soon after the resuscitation. Thus,
most times when the patient reaches the point where the
question of no code is raised, the decision whether to code
or not is a nondecision which has little effect on the
overall outcome. It only changes the specific time and
perhaps the mode of death.

However, even though the decision may in fact be not
as important as we make it out to be, it seems to be necessary in many cases. It is necessary because the nurses
require it as guidance, administrators want it for legal
reasons, and the lay public want it because they feel that
it is in fact a very crucial decision. Once the conclusion
that resuscitation is not indicated is reached, Rabkin
(Rabkin, Gillerman, Rice 1979) would insist that the final
decision should be made only by the informed consent of a
competent patient, or in the case of an incompetent patient,
the consent of all the family members. I think that, whenever possible, that is a very good idea. All physicians
making such decisions would prefer to have the blessings of
the patient, in particular and/or the family in these
situations. However, I take exception with whether or not
we call call it informed consent. This is a very important
matter. Let's take a situation like we have in this case.
Picture our patient, on a mechanical ventilator, plugged
into multiple intravenous lines, a Foley catheter draining
her urine, a feeding tube in her mouth, and a tube in her
throat so she can't talk. All she can do is shake her
head, and perhaps point to a letter on a board if she is so
able. You explain to her that her situation is hopeless,
there is no way we can alter the outcome, that if there is
any additional manipulation she is likely to have more pain
and more discomfort. Then you ask her if she agrees that
continued extraordinary care is no longer warranted. How

do you determine in this case whether the patient is even
competent to respond to such a question? This is a patient
who is under sedation, who is receiving analgesics, who's
been in an intensive care unit for 2 1/2 months where night
and day no longer have any meaning. Is she really competent
to make these kinds of decisions? Or, if you decide she is
not competent, you might approach her husband. In this
case, her husband was obviously unable to face the situation.
He was unable to even bear seeing her anymore, and unable or
unwilling to speak with physicians. You could, however, force
a confrontation and tell him the same thing. Your wife is
dying, she is suffering, we ask you for your informed consent not to resuscitate her the next time she dies. Even
under the best of circumstances, with a competent patient
and an emotionally stable family, which we weren't dealing
with here, is it possible for the physician to present this
as a real freedom of choice decision? I would imagine that
sometimes it is but not often. This decision in fact belongs
to the physician, and while he can attempt to diffuse his
responsibility out into the community, to the family, or to
the patient, he really can't give up his primary place in
this drama of life and death. In addition, he can't insulate
himself from the consequences of such a decision. To try
and use the courts to gain immunity from such decisions is
at best impractical and most often offers the legal system
the chance to make decisions that are not within their competence. The courts, in fact, appear to have formally
removed themselves from this question, making a clear distinction between active and passive considerations; between
the withdrawal of life supports and no code decisions. In
the Dinnerstein case in Massachusetts, the courts said that
the decision to resuscitate is a peculiarly medical decision
and the courts should not be involved.

Therefore, I again raise the question of whether it is
ever reasonable for the physician to take it upon himself
to make what may in fact be a nondecision about the advisa-
bility of resuscitation when the patient is unable to
participate in the decision. Is it possible that on some
occasions it may be more unjustified for the physicians to
seek aquiescence with this decision by the family than to
make the decision himself? The physician's first duty is
to his patient, but when the outcome is inevitable, shouldn't
he also begin to think about the survivors? How often do
we psychologically damage a family by forcing them to make
a decision that will actually play no role in the final outcome?

If it is occasionally appropriate for the physician to
make the decison without the formal consent of the patient
or family, what options does he have for carrying out his
decision? He can still write a no code order. However,
in some hospitals the consent of the family or patient must
be obtained before such an order is valid. The alternative
approach is to leave the decision regarding resuscitation
ambiguous. One might actually argue that this may be an
appropriate decision regardless of the situation - since
in fact the ultimate decision how or whether to resuscitate
may depend on what is required at the moment. To force the
physician, or patient, or family to make a simple code or
no code decision, I would contend oversimplifies a complex
decision-making process and may result in an inappropriate
response to a medical emergency. For example, we may have
a patient in whom the only thing that is required is to
reconnect him to the ventilator. That is one degree of
resuscitation. Perhaps all we need to do is reconnect him
to the ventilator and suction his endotracheal tube to get
rid of a plug of mucous that is blocking the airway. That
is another degree of resuscitation. Perhaps we only need to
intubate him or just defibrillate his heart one or two times
to achieve normal physiological function. If these simple
things don't work we must then decide whether or not to go
further. At the bedside we must decide is this a patient
we also want to put a pacemaker into; do we want to give him
intracardiac drugs; do we want to put him on a heart/lung
machine? In actuality during most resuscitative efforts
the decision of how long and how far to go is always influenced by the underlying condition of the patient. We
approach the seventy year old patient with diffuse metastatic cancer who has a cardiac arrest very differently
from the fifty year old patient who has just had a simple
operative procedure. There is no way to regulate this sort
of thing because there are no set rules for this game.
Thus, perhaps something between a code and no code decision
may be the most ethical decision in many situations.

Let me summarize by saying that the inputs to the final
decision of whether or not to resuscitate a patient are very
complex and very difficult to define absolutely. I think an
attempt to codify them into a moral or legal formula is not
possible at this time, and may in fact never be. While the
patient and the family must be maximally involved in decision
making whenever it can be accomplished, it may not always
be appropriate or advisable. If these arguments sound

paternalistic, and I'm sure they do, I offer no excuses, since, medicine is by its nature a paternalistic profession. This relationship between a doctor and his patient and the reality that the physician may sometimes make the wrong decision is one that we have to live with. However, until we reach the point where medical diagnoses and treatment can be reduced to the numbers 0 and 1 in a computer, it is likely to remain this way.

REFERENCES.

Rabkin MT, Gillerman G, Rice NR (1976). Orders not to resuscitate. N Engl J Med 295:364.
Veatch RM (1976). Death, dying and the biological revolution. New Haven: Yale University Press.
Lerner M (1970). When, why and where people die. In Brim OG(ed):"The Dying Patient," New York: Russell Sage Foundation, p 21.
Relman A (1979). Response to Buchanan. Am J Law and Med. 5:119.
Buchanan A (1979). Medical paternalism or legal imperialism. Am J Law and Med 5:97.

Troubling Problems in Medical Ethics: The Third
Volume in a Series on Ethics, Humanism, and Medicine: 141-142
© 1981 Alan R. Liss, Inc., 150 Fifth Ave., New York, NY 10011

DISCUSSION SUMMARY: THE DECISION TO RESUSCITATE - SLOWLY

Marc D. Basson
Director, CEHM
University of Michigan
Ann Arbor, Michigan

Virtually all the discussants believed that the ward
team should have tried harder to discuss Mrs. Sterling's
prognosis with her and her family before she became intermittently confused and before her impending death became
obvious. They argued that this would have made euthanasia
easier to discuss later and also that this would have given
the doctors some idea of the Sterlings' desires in this
regard. Even at the final decision point depicted in the
case, most discussants felt that more of an effort should
have been made to talk with the patient.

However, many discussants were disturbed by the external
factors (cost, intensive care unit space, hospital staff
time) which seemed strong arguments for allowing this woman
to die. There was a great deal of debate over whether it
was appropriate for the individual physician to consider
such factors in his decision making. Ultimately, about half
of the conference participants stated that it was wrong for
the physician to allow such considerations to come between
him and his patient. They therefore endorsed the University
of Michigan hospital policy prohibiting no code status
without the consent of the patient or his next of kin. They
further disapproved of any attempt at slow coding.

The other half of the discussants concluded that even
if the matter were discussed with Mr. Sterling and he wanted
"everything possible done", then it would still be wrong of
the doctors to undertake extraordinary resuscitative efforts
if Mrs. Sterling's heart stopped. (Indeed, they commented,
it might even be wrong of the physician to continue anti-

biotics and expensive electrolyte monitoring since these
will not change Mrs. Sterling's prognosis or keep her alive
for more than a few days while these efforts would waste
money that could be more effectively spent on other patients.)
If cost-effectiveness and considerations of scarce medical
resources require that the patient be allowed to die, some
participants argued, then it would indeed be, as Mrs. Sterling's
physician had written on her chart, "needless cruelty" to
ask Mr. Sterling if he would be willing to accept the guilt
of deciding for her death.

Of the half who felt that Mrs. Sterling would have to
be allowed to die regardless of her wishes or those of her
husband, most were seriously disturbed by the prospect of
lying to the Sterlings, for a slow code seemed fundamentally
dishonest. About half felt that the hospital policy was
wrong and should be changed. They would have preferred to
be able to tell the family that nothing further could be
done, allow them time to grieve and to say goodbye, and
then to abandon further resuscitative therapy. They stated
that if the hospital policy remained in force then the
external cost considerations gave the physician no choice
but to carry out a slow code.

The other 25% endorsed the needless cruelty argument and
felt that an unofficial slow code was appropriate for cases
such as that of Mrs. Sterling. They feared that if a policy
of making such patients "no code" without consent became a
matter of public record then patients' trust in their physician
would be destroyed. Slow codes, on the other hand, could by
their very nature easily be kept secret.

Seventh Conference on
Ethics, Humanism, and Medicine
March 21, 1981

**Troubling Problems in Medical Ethics: The Third
Volume in a Series on Ethics, Humanism, and Medicine: 145–149
© 1981 Alan R. Liss, Inc., 150 Fifth Ave., New York, NY 10011**

INTRODUCTION TO THE SEVENTH CONFERENCE: APPROACHES TO ETHICS

Marc D. Basson
Director, CEHM
University of Michigan
Ann Arbor, Michigan

Good morning and welcome to the Seventh Conference on
Ethics, Humanism and Medicine.

I hope that those who have attended these conferences
before have profited from them, and that all of you here today do the same. I know that I have learned a great deal over
the last four years, not only about medical ethics per se but
also about what it means to ask a question in medical ethics
and then to try to answer it. For the last six conferences
I told you that you must make up your own minds and that I
have no wish to persuade you to the views I express in my
opening remarks. Today I make no such disclaimers. I want
instead to talk about the philosophy underlying our conference
structure and the way I believe medical ethics ought to be
approached. This will be a brief excursion into metamedical
ethics, if you will forgive the phrase. I will oversimplify
grossly, but I hope the key points will come through.

If you listen to the discussion in your small group
today, or indeed to any ethical debate, you will notice that
the participants seem to argue in different ways. I'm not
talking about the different sorts of claims they make,
whether they support the right to privacy or oppose it. I'm
concerned rather with the way they advance their ethical
claims and the manner in which they support them. I want to
talk today about four ways to justify moral judgments.

The most primitive approach to ethical questions is one
I shall call intuitionism. This is the belief that an ethical
problem is not susceptible to logical analysis. One simply

thinks about the case and awaits a "gut reaction" or moral
intuition. The intuitionist approach need be neither simple-
minded nor insensitive. An intuitionist may extract and
weigh all the morally relevant facts before making a decision.
What distinguishes the intuitionist is what happens when you
ask him to justify his decision. Unable to articulate any
sort of general moral principle underlying his decision, the
intuitionist is reduced to restating key facts more loudly
and more emotionally.

To some extent we all rely on our moral intuitions
because we frequently lack the time or sophistication to
think through to the more general moral principles that
motivate us. I urge you, however, to recognize intuitionism
as a dangerous shortcut which ought to be avoided when possible. An unarticulated ethical stance cannot really be
analyzed, and the risk of ethical error is therefore high.

The mainstream metaethical notion I shall call absolutism is often presented as the major alternative to intuitionism. The ethical absolutist believes that every particular
moral judgment should be the conclusion of a syllogism with
premises including more general moral principles and observations about the case at hand. I suspect most of you
remember syllogisms, but briefly they are arguments from
stated premises to a logically entailed conclusion. For
instance, a well-known medical student syllogism: Anything
related to uric acid metabolism is boring. Gout is a defect
in uric acid metabolism. Therefore gout is boring.

The ethical absolutist applies this sort of argument
to moral questions. For instance, we might begin with the
general moral premise that it is wrong for a doctor to kill
a patient except when the patient is terminally ill, in
great pain, and asking to be killed. Coupled with the
factual premises that Mr. H is terminally ill, in great pain,
and asking to be killed, this logically implies that it may
be morally permissible for Mr. H's doctor to kill him. Of
course, general moral principles may also be attacked. One
might ask our imaginary moral absolutist why he thinks it
acceptable to kill people even when they are terminal and in
agony. He would then be compelled to offer us an even more
general moral principle and syllogism to support this judgment. (For instance: The doctor's prime duty is to prevent
needless suffering. A dying patient who no longer profits
from life is suffering needlessly. Therefore, the doctor

may kill him.)

This particular debate can and does run on forever. My point is that ethical absolutism, unlike intuitionism, permits us to carry on a cogent ethical argument. If two absolutists disagree, then they believe either that one has made an error in logic or that one syllogism begins with an incorrect factual or moral premise. Since these premises too must be the product of syllogistic reasoning, they are also vulnerable to analysis in their turn.

The biggest problem with moral absolutism is that some-times it doesn't seem possible to settle ethical disagreements in the way proposed. Antiabortionists say that killing humans is wrong and that the fetus is human. Therefore, abortion is wrong. Proabortionists say that killing humans is wrong only after they have reached some degree of gestational maturity and that clearly some fetuses have not reached this level. Therefore, they conclude that aborting these fetuses is permissible. The argument escalates in complexity rapidly (at least for those antiabortionists willing to engage in logical analysis) and yet despite the efforts of some superb philosophers we are left with two irreconcilable sets of moral principles, one favoring abortion and one opposing it. There does not seem to be any mutually accepted general moral principle which the two sides might use to adjudicate between their views.

Ethical relativism represents a reaction to this diffi-culty. The ethical relativist says that the proabortionists and antiabortionists can't find a moral principle in common because none exists. Neither is wrong, the relativist claims. It is just that abortion is wrong for Mrs. X (an antiabortion-ist) even though it might be permissible for Mrs. Y (a pro-abortionist) in the same circumstances.

While the ethical relativist believes in general moral principles and syllogistic ethical analysis, he does not believe that his general moral principles are necessarily generalizable to other people. Moral argument is meaningful for the relativist only when the two participants share moral premises and can therefore compare logic. To the extent to which one is a relativist one is likely to quit when an ethical debate gets tough and to attribute the disagreement to un-resolvable differences in intuition rather than faulty logic or improperly derived premises. Relativism preserves the

machinery of absolutist ethical debate but removes most of
its motivation.

Ethical absolutism seems an almost impossible view given
the seemingly unresolvable quality of debates such as that
over abortion. In addition, it has historically led to great
excesses by zealots and fanatics. The Spanish Inquisitors,
the Crusaders, the Nazis, all were in their own way ethical
absolutists acting out nightmarish moral codes. Ethical
relativism enables us to explain irreconcilable moral
differences while preserving the possibility of moral argument, but it also undercuts the very purpose of ethical
debate. After all, we want not only to decide what we
ought to do but also to convince others to act rightly. We
want to be able to say that the Nazis and the Spanish In-
quistors were wrong no matter what they believed and no
matter what cultural heritage produced them.

The solution lies in ethical pluralism. The ethical
pluralist begins with two assumptions. First, he accepts
the basic premise of absolutism, that universalizable moral
principles exist. Second, he recognizes that he cannot always
deduce these moral principles with certainty, that it is hard
to apply them and even harder to convince others of them.

From these premises, the pluralist moves to the conclusion that under some circumstances he ought to tolerate the
beliefs and actions of others even if he believes them
ethically improper. He may reach this conclusion by a de-
ontologic argument from rights of privacy, via a moral
principle to the effect that one ought not to force others
to commit one's own errors, or because of consequentialist
arguments from the counterproductivity of endless bickering.
I have not time to work these arguments through here. Rather
let me conclude by sketching briefly the implications of the
pluralist view. The pluralist believes his moral judgments
are right, but recognizes that they may be wrong. He acts
on the basis of his own conclusions even when he risks great
wrong, for his reasoning is the best he has to go on. On
the other hand, because he recognizes (albeit doubtfully)
that he might be in error the pluralist does not generally
force his ethical beliefs on others. In extreme cases, such
as the Inquisition or Nazi Party, he may find that the strength
of his conviction outweighs his uncertainty and that the
gravity of the moral crimes overshadows the prima facie
pluralistic principle. In these cases, the pluralist is

prepared to act on his convictions.

The ethical pluralist is crucially different from the ethical relativist. The relativist denies the interpersonal universalizability of moral judgments. He may attempt ethical debate but ultimately he must acknowledge that the other's view is as right as his own. The pluralist, on the other hand, takes as an article of faith that all moral debates have resolutions, if only we had time and wit enough to find them. While the relativist accepts disagreement over ethical questions, the pluralist merely tolerates it.

This is the attitude I wish to urge upon you and which CEHM has been established to foster. You will find great diversity in your small group discussions today, and even more out in the real world. In addition to learning something about the topics you will hear discussed today, I hope that you will practice conducting logical ethical arguments with those who disagree. By the end of the small group discussions, some of you will have managed to persuade or be persuaded by others with whom you disagreed initially. Persuaders or persuaded, you will have successfully participated in an ethical debate, a debate whose true purpose is not to persuade but to establish moral truth. Others of you will end your discussions as you began, unpersuaded and apparently not successfully persuasive. If you fall into this category, then you will have an opportunity to practice something even more valuable, the attitude of pluralism. Remember that if I fail to convince you and you fail to convince me, this does not mean that we are both right (although we may both be wrong). Instead, it means that we lack the skill to mount an ethical debate sufficiently sophisticated to resolve our disagreement. The solution is to keep practicing until we get there, but to live and work with each other in the meantime.

Troubling Problems in Medical Ethics: The Third Volume in a Series on Ethics, Humanism, and Medicine: 151–152
© **1981 Alan R. Liss, Inc., 150 Fifth Ave., New York, NY 10011**

INTRODUCTION: COMPETENCE AND THE RIGHT TO REFUSE TREATMENT

Rachel Lipson
Program Director, CEHM
University of Michigan
Ann Arbor, Michigan

What happens when a patient refuses treatment? His wishes are usually honored since few would argue against the right of a competent adult to refuse treatment. However, the competence of a patient may often be in doubt in such situations, and if a person is judged incompetent, he may lose his right to make decisions regarding his own health care.

What do we mean when we say a patient is competent to consent to or to refuse treatment? In a recent paper in the Journal of Medical Ethics, Elias Baumgarten explains that the competent patient is "generally entitled to a large measure of control over medical decisions that will affect him." (Baumgarten, 1980). Such a person presumably has the mental capacity to understand the medical information necessary to make such decisions, and is reasonable enough to use this information to best achieve his goals. (Courts have ruled that a patient may refuse treatment for any reason, even if it seems bizarre, so long as he appears to understand the consequences of his choice.) But who is to judge whether a patient is capable of integrating medical information about his case into a reasonable decision?

Edward Goldman examines the legal system's role in deciding whether a patient is competent to refuse treatment. He points out that the question of proper treatment is often subsumed under the issue of who decides competency, for if the patient is judged incompetent, the court is free to appoint a guardian who favors treatment. Goldman questions the morality of such court decisions and concludes his paper by stressing that the courts' bias should be toward judging

the patient competent rather than against this. Goldman
feels that the health care team should not use judgments
of incompetence as a means of forcing treatment upon patients.

In addition, Goldman enumerates seven groups of people
who may decide whether the patient is competent, and analyses
the strengths and weaknesses of each possibility. He also
examines the notion of competence in legal terms and points
out that there are at least a dozen different kinds of competence recognized by law. Each sort of competence is
defined by different rules motivated by different underlying
issues. Thus, when we evaluate competence we must always ask
what it is that we are judging the patient competent to do.
An individual may be competent to perform one sort of action
but not another.

Dr. Robert Sadoff emphasizes the importance of the
manner in which the doctor presents factual information to
the patient, reminding us that sometimes it is the professional
rather than the patient who is incompetent. Sadoff also
considers the practical question of how a psychiatrist
evaluates a given patient's competence. Sadoff describes
the mental status exam he performs when he interviews a
patient to determine if the patient is capable of giving
consent for treatment. He also reminds us that the patient's
emotional state may affect the patient's ability to make
reasonable decisions. An understanding of the socio-
cultural framework in which the patient lives may also be
important. Sadoff suggests that the physician should have a
set of routine questions that he always uses to evaluate
competence, and that he should not let preconceived biases
interfere with this process, for the person who seems incompetent at first glance is not necessarily so. Sadoff
ends his discussion by considering Norman Cousins's "The
Anatomy of an Illness as Perceived by the Patient," and
comments on the implications of Cousins's story for the
physician-patient interaction.

REFERENCE

Baumgarten E (1980). The concept of "competence" in medical
    ethics. J Med Ethics 6:180.

Troubling Problems in Medical Ethics: The Third
Volume in a Series on Ethics, Humanism, and Medicine: 153–155
© **1981 Alan R. Liss, Inc., 150 Fifth Ave., New York, NY 10011**

COMPETENCE AND THE RIGHT TO REFUSE TREATMENT

CASE FOR DISCUSSION

Arthur Millburn, a 91 year old ex-bricklayer with a history of severe congestive heart failure currently controlled on diuretics, was brought to University Hospital by his daughter. She complained that he had been having severe diarrhea and constant fecal incontinence for the past month. He was also found to have chronic urinary incontinence. At the time of admission, he could identify his name, the hospital, and the day of the week. He recalled only one of three objects at 2 minutes, however, and was four years off on the current year. He refused further mental status testing because he did not want to made fun of. He had been living with his daughter and her family for the last five years.

A one week workup revealed a large premalignant colonic polyp (a villous adenoma) which was probably causing the diarrhea. Benign prostatic hypertrophy was identified as the cause of urinary incontinence. The polyp (which was not cancerous but had approximately a 20% chance of becoming so in the future) was too large to be removed endoscopically. Millburn's options were therefore either to undergo surgery with a small but real risk of complications or death, or to leave the polyp alone, live with his diarrhea, and hope that the polyp did not grow to obstruct his bowel. (This would require emergency surgery with a high mortality rate.) The doctors were unable to promise Millburn that removing the polyp would cure his diarrhea, but they believed that this would work. The urologists, who had been consulted about Millburn's urinary problems, recommended that he undergo a transurethral resection of his prostate (TURP). This procedure, which is done through the penile urethra without an incision, offered a 50% chance of improving Millburn's urinary incontinence with only a small chance of worsening the problem. A TURP could either be done during the same anesthetic as the polypectomy or under spinal anesthesia without the risks of putting Millburn to sleep.

The intern taking care of Millburn explained these findings and options to him and recommended that he undergo a TURP and operative polypectomy. The intern told Millburn that the abdominal and urologic surgeons would come by later to tell him more about the risks and benefits of these procedures. Millburn replied, "I'm an old man and I can't remember things people tell me all the time, but if this will fix my water and bowels, then that's what I want."

When the surgeons told him that these procedures could result in death, however, Millburn changed his mind. "I ain't about to let no one operate on me and kill me," he explained to his intern afterwards. "They told me I might die!"

However, Mr. Millburn's daughter, who worked as a ward clerk on the surgical floor, insisted that he undergo surgery. "Dad's got problems and you can fix them," she said. "He's been unbearable lately. Besides you're telling me that the polyp might turn into a cancer some day. It should be taken out." She talked with Millburn the next day and triumphantly returned to the ward team with the news that Millburn had consented to surgery. The surgeons were reconsulted, but by the time they arrived two days later Millburn was once again refusing surgery.

Discussion of how to treat Millburn went on for two more weeks. He was recolonoscoped twice so that staff surgeons could see the polyp for themselves and decide whether they thought they could remove it through the colonoscope. (They could not.) His diarrhea was further aggravated by the enemas he received before each procedure and he became steadily more miserable.

Millburn was approached several more times regarding possible consent to surgery, by his daughter, by the ward team, and by the surgeons. These encounters sometimes resulted in consent, and other times in emphatic refusal. He freqently brushed off his doctors' questions with "I'll do

whatever my daughter thinks best. You just go and ask her."
When his daughter would talk with him, Millburn would agree,
but the surgeons who were then called would either fail to
obtain consent or (in two instances) successfully obtained
consent only to have Millburn forget that he had given it
and refuse to enter the operating suite.

Millburn became increasingly disoriented and apathetic.
By his fourth week in the hospital, he spoke only in short
phrases and only when prompted. He refused most of his
food. When the nurses attempted to feed him, he would
repeat over and over, "I'm just an old man. All I want to
do is die. Why don't you let me die?" He no longer re-
membered what day or season it was and frequently could not
remember that he was in a hospital. He was unable to remember having talked to someone five minutes earlier.

The daughter insisted that all steps should be taken to
"fix Dad up like new." She vowed to convince her father at
all costs. Millburn's nurse, who had worked in a nursing
home previously, had reservations. "Arthur is competent to
make his own decisions," she contended, "or at least he was
when he came in here and refused surgery. He told me that
just last month he had his driver's license renewed and his
daughter tells me he rewrote his will a few months ago.
I've seen an elderly patient's competence doubted too many
times when he didn't want something the doctors did and they
pushed him into it."

Was Mr. Millburn competent to refuse surgery at the
beginning of his hospitalization? Should he have been sent
home when he refused? Would it have been appropriate, as
one physician suggested, to declare him incompetent at the
end of the case and let his daughter sign the operative
permits? What criteria are necessary or sufficient for
determining the competence to accept or refuse treatment?
What do we mean by competence?

(Case prepared by Mary Fox and Marc D. Basson.)

Troubling Problems in Medical Ethics: The Third
Volume in a Series on Ethics, Humanism, and Medicine: 157-167
© 1981 Alan R. Liss, Inc., 150 Fifth Ave., New York, NY 10011

COMPETENCY AND THE RIGHT TO REFUSE TREATMENT: WHO'S IN
CHARGE?

Edward B. Goldman

Hospital Attorney
University of Michigan
Ann Arbor, Michigan 48109

INTRODUCTION

    I will view this case from the perspective of the legal
system. Issues that the law has to resolve will be discussed
followed by a brief review of several decided cases and then
a discussion of the specific questions raised by our hypothetical case.

UNDERLYING ISSUES FOR THE LEGAL SYSTEM

    Two basic issues clash in this area: the principle of
freedom and self-determination in life and death issues versus a compelling interest in the preservation of human life.

    The self-determination case is well stated by John Ste-
wart Mills in his essay "On Liberty" when he asserts that the
only purpose for which power can be rightfully exercised over
a member of a civilized community against his will is to prevent harm to others. An individual's own good is not a sufficient warrant.

    The notion of a compelling interest in preserving human
life is known in the law as "parens patriae", a Latin term
meaning the state shall assume the role and authority of a
parent. For example, the state can compel blood transfusions
for children of Jehovah's Witnesses. In non-medical areas
the state for the child's welfare can remove children from
parents in divorce or abuse and neglect cases. Why should
the same benevolent rule not apply to adults?

The legal system's basic rule is that competent adults can not be compelled to accept treatment against their will. The key question then becomes the definition of competence.

COMPETENCY: WHAT IS IT?

A brief definition: competency is a legal status that allows an individual to control what happens to the individual's person or property.

The law has developed notions of competency in a fragmented way and currently at least one dozen different types of competency are analyzed by the law. Each type has slightly different underlying issues and slightly different rules for resolution. A few brief examples will show the different items focused on by the legal system.

1. Competency to Make a Will.

Necessary items included are: legal age of majority, ability to know nature and extent of property, ability to recall natural objects of bounty, and ability to determine and understand disposition of property. The underlying issue is that the person making the will has an intact memory and has not been subject to fraud or undue influence in determining how the property is to be transferred.

2. Competency to Marry.

Necessary statuses include minimum age and avoidance of violating societal rules against incest or marriage between close relatives. Underlying issues include genetic concerns, society's view of morality and a certain minimum age as evidence of sound judgment.

3. Competency to Stand Trial.

Necessary status is an ability to provide information to and effectively assist defense attorney at trial. The underlying issue is the legal system's concern that the trial be fair and that the defendant have a chance to understand the case brought against the defendant and be able to effectively assist in the case's defense.

4. Competency to Have a Driver's License.

Necessary status is minimum age and adequate motor skills, judgment skills, and knowledge of traffic rules. The underlying issue is one of safety for other drivers and pedestrians.

5. Competency to Practice a Profession (or a Skill).

Necessary status is a certain level of education and a demonstration of good moral conduct and knowledge of requisite professional skills. This is generally determined by a standardized test (for example the exams given in law or medicine). Underlying issue is protection of other members of society from incompetent professionals. This applies equally to driving a car or using a scalpel.

The above brief examples are areas well worked out in the law. The question of "competency to refuse treatment" is a newcomer to the law and does not have the same detailed legal history and attention. Courts and legislatures have normally said that competency to refuse treatment is based on the ability of the patient to understand the nature and consequences of the patient's actions. A competent patient may refuse treatment for a mere whim. The patient needs only to understand and not to justify the refusal in almost all cases. This area does not seek to define property rights (right to give away money, drive car, practice law) but rather looks to control over the patient's body. In a few cases courts have refused to follow the general rule on competency to refuse treatment because they feel a more fundamental right is at stake. In two adult Jehovah Witnesses cases, courts have ordered competent adults to undergo treatment on the rationale that their refusal resulting in death would make their children wards of the state. Thus, the court orders treatment in order to avoid harm to the children. See Application of President and Directors of Georgetown College, Inc. 32 Ill 2d 361, 205 NE 2d 435 (1965) and Raleigh Fitkin-Paul Morgan Memorial Hospital v. Anderson 42 NJ 421, 201 A 2d 537 (1964). And, in one case, Commissioner of Corrections v. Meyers _____ NY _____ (1979); a competent prisoner was ordered to undergo dialysis treatment even though he refused. The court held to allow the refusal would allow the patient to die before his sentence had been served and therefore would fail to uphold the integrity of the prison system. With these very few exceptions, the rule is well established that a competent patient may refuse treatment and that refusal must be respected.

Thus, the stated legal idea is that a <u>competent</u> patient is in control. Michigan law says this is so important that a finding of mental illness and involuntary civil commitment is not equal to a loss of competency. So, a patient can be committed to a mental institution and still retain the right to make contracts, make wills, have a driver's license, and run for political office. MCLA 300.1702. However, in practice some courts have focused on the patient's decision and its results rather than on the patient's ability to understand. In other words, some courts may be paying lip service to the standard then interpreting the facts to achieve a result the judges - rather than the patient - desire.

SUICIDE: A SIDE ISSUE

Some argument has been made that any refusal of treatment is suicide which is either illegal, immoral, or at least in bad taste.

Courts have easily resolved this issue by saying that letting nature take its course without active intervention is not suicide. So, while it is theoretically possible to use this argument to justify an order compelling treatment, courts with very rare exceptions have found the argument not to be compelling. See Veatch (1976) <u>Death, Dying and the Biological Revolution: A Last Quest for Responsibility</u>, Chapter 4.

This provides no easy out and the issue of competency must be squarely addressed.

WHO DECIDES COMPETENCY?

Since we know that a competent patient is in charge, the important issue becomes who decides that the patient is competent and on what basis is the decision made.

A Broadway play entitled "Whose Life Is It Anyway" poses who decides as the play's central issue. The central character is a young patient paralyzed from the neck down. The patient, a sculptor now unable to work, is kept alive by medical treatment and seeks to have the treatment discontinued. The play dramatically and forcefully argues that the legal bias should be strongly in favor of the patient's autonomy. In one brief example, a physician wants to give the patient Valium and the patient responds that if the patient makes the physician uneasy, that's the physician's problem and the physician should take the Valium.

In analyzing the question of who decides competency, cases have looked at the following possibilities:
1. The patient.
2. The physician. Of course, the physician may feel the patient is being irrational by refusing treatment and therefore say any patient refusing treatment must be incompetent. Or, the physician could be feeling rejected and impotent and therefore try to show that the patient is incompetent.
3. An uninvolved psychiatric consultation. It is unclear whether a consultant can truly be uninvolved and whether a consultant will use standards acceptable to the legal system.
4. The courts. Physicians have argued that judges do not understand medicine and the court system is a cumbersome method of resolving medical questions.
5. The family. Problems arise deciding who represents the family where views are split and deciding whether the family has an interest contrary to the patient's interest. For example, do family members stand to inherit if the patient dies?
6. An ethics committee of the hospital composed of physicians and lay persons. Problems around this group include lack of adequate knowledge about the patient and being so neutral that they cannot truly be interest in the individual patient's welfare.
7. A person named in a living will by the patient. This is an idea of substituted consent where the patient when competent can self-appoint a guardian and set conditions that the guardian must follow. For example, the patient can name a close friend as a guardian and state that no heroic measures should be employed to prolong life. This has been criticized on the basis that patients when healthy cannot really imagine what their views will be once they become ill.

Resolving the issue of who decides competency often resolves the treatment issue. If a patient is found incompetent by the court then the court is free to appoint an individual who is known to be in favor of treatment and will therefore give consent.

This leaves the question of whether the system should encourage a decision that the patient is incompetent so some

treatment can be given or at least a third party appointed
by the court can make decisions about treatment.

THE BASIS FOR A DECISION ON COMPETENCY

In arriving at an operational definition of competency,
courts have looked, at least, at the following factors without any detailed attempt to quantify the relative importance
of each:
1. Medical status.
2. Age.
3. Patient's value to society.
4. The future quality of the patient's life. Will
treatment extend life for a brief period or will it be cura-
tive?
5. Patient's desires as can be determined from patient
or third parties who are familiar with patient's desires.
6. Desires of the family.
7. Desires of the physician to treat or refrain from
treating.
8. Cost benefit analysis on a theory of whether it is
unduly costly to preserve vegetative individuals in costly
Intensive Care Unit beds.
9. Overall societal values dealing with preservation of
life.

Clearly in examining these areas courts are deviating
from the basic rule of simply determining whether the patient
is competent. Thus, to some extent, judges are imposing
their own values on the decision to allow treatment.

CASE LAW EXAMPLES

This section will discuss several cases and attempt to
place them in logical rather than chronological order.

In Re: Brown 45 Mich 326 (1881). An 80 year old individual provided for his food, shelter, and burial and then
began giving away his other money. His family sued to have
him declared incompetent so they could take over handling
of his funds. The court after determining that the individual had taken care of all of his necessary needs felt that he
may be unwise but this was not equal to incompetency.

Religion Cases. In a number of Christian Scientist
and Jehovah Witness cases involving adults, courts have held

that adults may refuse treatment based on religious grounds.
See for example In the Matter of Melideo 390 NYS 2d 523 (1976).

In Re: Quackenbush No. F3-1483 NJ Super Jan 13, 1978.
Here a conscious alert patient refused surgery to remove his
gangrenous leg. The patient had diabetes and had not properly cared for himself. The court ordered an examination and
found that the patient understood the nature of his illness
and that death would ensue if he refused treatment. Since
the patient understood the consequences, the court found him
competent and refused to allow surgery.

In Re: Eisner (Brother Fox) 73 A.D. 2d 431 N.Y. (1981).
Here the patient was unconscious but had been a member of a
monastery for a number of years and his views on preservation
of life were well known to the other members of the monastery.
They testified that Brother Fox had strongly held convictions
against being placed on a respirator or having extraordinary
measures taken to prolong life. The court found that if
Brother Fox were conscious he would refuse further treatment
and held treatment could be discontinued.

In Re: Quinlan 70 N.J. 10 (1976). Here the patient
was in a non-reversible extended persistent vegatative state.
However, as opposed to Brother Fox, Karen Quinlan's views
were not established. The court had to engage in guesswork
to determine whether she wanted treatment continued. The
court said "if Karen Ann were miraculously competent but
with the same medical condition, she would ask for the machines to be turned off". Since no evidence of her views existed, this appears to be more guesswork than knowledge on
the court's part and may be a case of the court substituting
its feelings for those of the patient where the patient's
condition is hopeless.

In Re: Carrie Ann McNaulty (Discussed in Holder, Legal
Issues in Pediatrics and Adolescent Medicine. Massachusetts
trial court decision.) Here a mentally retarded child was
born with a cardiac defect. The defect could be repaired
but the child was felt to be seriously mentally retarded and
would have to spend her life in an institution since the parents were unwilling to have her at home. Parents refused
consent for the surgery and the surgeons agreed. Because of
the Quinlan case and because of the hospital's desire to be
sure that a proper course was being followed in accepting
the parent's refusal, the case went to court. In this case

since McNaulty was a newborn her views could not be known.
But, because McNaulty's condition was treatable, the court
held that the parent's refusal of consent would not be honored
and that the surgeons must treat the child. The court may
have been saying that if McNaulty could talk, unlike Quinlan,
she would say go ahead and treat. Alternatively, the court
may have focused solely on the fact that McNaulty's condition
was reversible while Quinlan's was not.

In general then, the cases resolve the issue of who decides competency by saying that the court will decide. It
then resolves the question of the basis for the decision by
looking at medical testimony, patient's ability to knowingly
refuse treatment and for comatose patients, the patient's
desires as the court can determine them. If an alert patient
clearly does not desire treatment and understands the consequences of refusal, courts tend to honor that refusal. If
the patient is incompetent and the condition is uncorrectable,
untreatable, and terminal within a short defined period of
time, the courts will not generally order treatment. A common example is end stage amyotrophic lateral sclerosis (Lou
Gehrig's Disease) an untreatable irreversible neurological
condition. If patient's desires are not known, but the condition is treatable, courts generally order treatment.

ISSUES RAISED BY THE HYPOTHETICAL CASE

Lawyers tend to look for cases exactly on point since
these serve as precedent and perhaps also as an excuse for
detailed intellectual analysis. There are two on point cases
similar to our hypothetical case. Unfortunately they come
out with contradictory results.

In the first case a 67 year old with gangrene of the
right foot is examined by three psychiatrists who agree that
the patient lacks capacity to understand the nature of the
physical condition and the need for amputation. The court
finds the patient incompetent and appoints as guardian a
family member who will consent to treatment. In the Matter
of William Schiller 148 NJ Supra 168; 372 A 2d 360 (1977).

The second case: In Petition of Nemser 51 Mich 2d 616;
273 NYS 2d 624 (1966) concerns an 80 year old widow with
gangrene of the foot who is examined and is felt not to be
competent. However, the woman has three children two of whom
are in favor of amputation while the third - a physician -

is opposed. The court ducks the issue of competency and treatment by saying that since the family members are not in agreement and since the physician is opposed, it does not appear that surgery is a matter of life and death and therefore the court will not order surgery.

The issues raised by our hypothetical case include at least the following items for small group discussion:

1. Is our patient more like Quinlan or McNaulty? Is the patient's medical condition non-reversible? In this case, the polyp is said to be easily treatable. Is the patient' senility irreversible? Perhaps, but that is not the condition to be treated. Also, the patient may have senility (insufficient blood flow to the brain on occasion) or may simply be lonely, suffering from malnutrition, or suffering from infection. If this is the case, the condition can be corrected and perhaps the patient can be made more competent.

2. Is the patient really refusing treatment? At times the patient does seem to consent while at other times he balks. Is this based on how the material is presented to the patient? For example, could there be a different result if the physicians had deemphasized the risk of death or had presented the case for surgery to the patient in a more sympathetic light?

3. Does old age in and of itself equal incompetence? If not, should we take into account the daughter's feelings of frustration at having to take care of her father. In other words, who do we define as the patient?

Perhaps because the patient is 91 years old and has a severe heart condition it may be better to leave him alone than put him under the stress of surgery. If so, should this decision be made by the daughter, physician, court, or the patient and how should it be presented to the patient?

4. Can the daughter obtain consent for the doctors? The daughter is a ward clerk familiar with the risks, benefits, and alternatives to the surgical procedure and reported to the surgeon that her father had consented. Why not go ahead on the basis that she has obtained consent? If the physician's only concern is the possibility of a later lawsuit, the 91 year old is unlikely to sue and the daughter having obtained consent would have a difficult time bringing a lawsuit based on lack of informed consent against the physician. Of course, this approach does not resolve the ethical issue and

is not even legally defensible but is it responsible for the
physician to be willing to assume the risk of suit and go a-
head with the surgery? In other words, is this civil dis-
obedience or simply flouting the law?

5. Did the lengthy hospital stay induce depression so
that the patient was initially competent but became incompetent? If so, can a physician bootstrap his or her way into
a finding that a patient is incompetent? For example, a physician could do a detailed note in the medical record stressing the patient's lack of cooperation, disorientation, and
inability to demonstrate adequate memory or insight. This
could be the basis for probate court to appoint a guardian
who could give consent to the surgical procedure.

In some cases physicians fairly routinely ignore patient
requests on the grounds that the patient is intermittently incompetent. For example, severely burned patients typically
ask that treatment be discontinued and they be allowed to die.
Burn Unit staff routinely ignore such requests on the grounds
that patient is not rational and is requesting death only because the pain is so severe. Could the physicians in this
case say the patient was competent when he gave initial consent and then became incompetent?

6. Would your opinion change if the patient had recently rewritten his will leaving nothing to his daughter who is
described in the will as ungrateful and instead leaving a
large amount of money to the University Hospital? Does this
present a conflict of interest which may render the physician's
decision not to treat suspect?

CONCLUSIONS

In analyzing these cases, I look at technical and policy
issues. I define technical issues as medical facts about the
patient's prognosis and options and policy issues as what
should be done given the patient's prognosis and options.

Physicians are well trained to provide an answer to the
technical questions and can and should provide options including preferred options and counselling. The counselling
should extend to the physician's view about what should be
done. However, the policy question on what should be done
should be answered by the patient and medicine and the legal
system should provide all necessary assistance to insure a
bias on the side of the patient being seen as competent.

Although it may be expedient in our case to present the
case to probate court in a way that the court will find the
patient incompetent and appoint the daughter to give approval for the treatment, I prefer sending the patient home
and allowing the patient to become reoriented.   Once this has
occurred, the patient can be approached by the physician in
a non-threatening way and can engage in detailed discussion
with the physician about the treatment in a less paternalistic fashion.   Benefit of the doubt should be on competency
and the health care team should make efforts to bolster
rather than undermine competency of a patient.   Equally the
legal system should favor and encourage patient self-determination.

**Troubling Problems in Medical Ethics: The Third
Volume in a Series on Ethics, Humanism, and Medicine: 169–176
© 1981 Alan R. Liss, Inc., 150 Fifth Ave., New York, NY 10011**

COMPETENCY AND THE RIGHT TO REFUSE TREATMENT

Robert L. Sadoff, M.D.
Department of Psychiatry
University of Pennsylvania
Suite 326, The Benjamin Fox Pavilion
Jenkintown, Pennsylvania

INTRODUCTION

I have prepared some very informal comments on competency.
I have three or four major outlined areas. The first is general background. I don't really think you can talk about
competency without talking about informed consent, since we
need to know whether the patient is competent to hear the
information given him and whether he is competent to give
consent. Ed Goldman asked the question "Who's in charge?"
Let me modify that. Instead of "Who's in charge?", let me
ask "Who is competent to decide?" That will give you some
idea of where I'm going to focus.

The patient is not the only one we are concerned about
in terms of competency. I have seen doctors who are incompetent to make the medical decisions they have made,
leading to damage to the patient. I have seen lawyers,
judges, and family members in all areas of competency issues
who were incompetent to make the decisions they made for the
patient also leading sometimes to tragic results.

INFORMED CONSENT

There are many different kinds of consent: vicarious,
presumed, implied, and informed. Informed consent is the
one we have to deal with and that includes such questions as
what we tell the patient and how much we tell him. How do
we tell the patient? Do we say, "You know if you have this
operation, buddy, you're going to die!" No, it is a very
artistic or artful manner of dealing with patients: how

much is told, how it is told, and what tone of voice is used. For example, in my practice of forensic psychiatry, very often I will be appointed by the prosecutor or the district attorney to examine a defendant in prison. I may go into the prison and say, "I'm Dr. Sadoff, I'm a psychiatrist. I've been asked to see you by the prosecutor. Now, what you tell me in the course of our interview, I'm going to put down on paper. I will put it into a letter that I'm going to send to the prosecutor who is going to use it to try to convict you of this charge. Do you still want to talk with me?" Usually the defendant feels fairly comfortable hearing that type of opening statement. He may feel that this is the first time anyone has been so open and above board with him.

But if a person goes in as some students may do and says in a very rote and rapid fashion, "I'm Dr. Jones and I'm here to ask you some questions at the request of the prosecutor and what you tell me I'm going to put into a report and he will use it to try to put you in jail"; then the defendant may say, "You can go to hell - I'm not going to talk with you." I would not blame them. It's a matter of how the material is presented, in what way and how sincerely it is presented, that determines whether the prisoner or the patient is willing to talk to the doctor.

THE RIGHT TO REFUSE TREATMENT

We've had some problems in psychiatry in assessing a patient's right to refuse treatment - usually the right to refuse medication. There are several recent cases that have made some impact in psychiatry. I raise these cases because they do have implications generally in medicine. You have to understand how the law has developed in this area. Ed Goldman mentioned involuntary commitment. If a patient is committed to a hospital against his will, doctors have argued to the patient when wishing to give medication against his will, "Look, the judge put you in here for treatment. I feel an obligation to treat you. Not only that, but the law has mandated, under the cases of Wyatt v. Stickney (1971), Rouse v. Cameron (1966), and Donaldson v. O'Connor (1974), that you have a constitutional right to treatment, and by God you are going to get it!"

That really isn't what the right to treatment says, and there are psychiatrists that have said when you offer someone the right to refuse treatment you give him "one right too many." I don't agree. I believe the right to refuse treatment is an integral part of the patient's right to adequate treatment. The treatment must be made available but not forced upon the patient against his will unless he is incompetent to decide or unless it is an emergency.

COMPETENCY

If the person is committed to the hospital is he generally competent to make decisions for himself? In the past, a person who was committed to the hospital was automatically deemed incompetent for various aspects of his life including managing his own affairs. At present such a patient is no longer deemed incompetent and has his rights intact. For example, he can vote. But that is a practical matter. How does a person in a hospital go to the polls and vote? There have to be people who are willing to take him if his polling place is far from the hospital. He also has the right to drive, but a question may be raised in terms of his privacy. If the doctor is putting a patient on heavy tranquilizing medication that might affect his three-dimensional vision or other aspects of his behavior and control, is this reported to the Motor Vehicles Division so the patient's license is lifted, or does he have a right to privacy so that such information is not given to deprive him of his right to drive? Driving may be seen as a privilege because other people's lives may be at stake if an incompetent person drives, or a person who is under heavy doses of medication. Nevertheless, there are some areas where such information may be provided without the patient's informed consent.

Another question is raised regarding the patient's competency within the hospital. Should the competency hearings be held at the time of the involuntary commitment? As you have heard, there are twelve different kinds of competency and I won't repeat them at this time, but the major issue here is the competency of the patient to determine his medical treatment and/or to refuse medication. Most courts have decided that the issue of competency is not to be decided at the time of commitment but at some later time. Doctors have encouraged the courts to make such a decision at the time of commitment so they can begin treatment immediately since that appears to be the purpose of involuntary hospitalization. One recent case proposed that a person who is committed to the hospital against his will is so committed because he cannot give a rational choice about his treatment; therefore, the notion is extended to the concept of his choice of medication as well as his choice of treatment in a hospital or in the community. That is just one case among many. Two other cases more clearly illustrate the patient's right to refuse medication. They are complex cases that reach substantially the same conclusion, but differ in two major respects: (a) Who decides competency and (b) Who decides whether the patient may refuse his medication?

In the Rogers (1979) case in Massachusetts, the judge decided that the determination of competency was a judicial matter; i.e., only a judge can decide. He also stated that only the judge, and not the psychiatrist, will decide who may refuse medication. On the other hand, the judge in the Rennie (1978) case in New Jersey stated that competency can be determined by the treating physician, labeling it "functional incompetency". The doctor may decide that a person is not competent to make the decision about his treatment and may go ahead and treat until the judge has the chance to hear the evidence in the matter. The judge in the Rennie case also allowed for a neutral psychiatrist to be appointed in lieu of the court to decide the medical issue of medical treatment for the patient.

PRACTICAL GUIDELINES FOR COMPETENCY EXAMINATIONS

What are the guidelines that I use to evaluate a person for competency to make decisions regarding his treatment? First of all, we do what is called a mental status examination. That is, we see what the person's orientation is. Can he focus on various things? Can he remember both short term and long term items? I usually ask the patient to recall three objects after five minutes. I may ask people what they had for lunch or dinner. I may ask about the patient's ability to concentrate by asking him to substract serial three's or seven's, depending on his intelligence. I also check on his ability to abstract by asking him to interpret well-known proverbs. These are the basic aspects of a mental status examination.

Secondly, I look at the psychology of the patient in terms of his mood. Is he depressed? Does he have anxiety which might reduce his ability to make judgments for himself? What are the family pressures? Who is in the family? Who will benefit from whether he is operated on or not? And, finally, what is his age?

Thirdly, I look at the socio-cultural aspects of his life. This is very important since I'm a white, middle class individual from the Mid-West who may be examining a person from a totally different culture. One example comes to mind. I had the experience of examining an Ethiopian man who had hijacked an airplane in Philadelphia and I thought he was incompetent. I didn't know enough about his background or his culture since I didn't speak Amheric, the language of Ethiopia. I started to read books on Ethiopia and to talk with other people from that country to find out whether or not what this man told me was culturally derived or whether it was psychotic. At the end, my opinion was that he was psychotic and that he was not competent to stand trial. He was tried anyway and found guilty. Thus, the judge does not always agree with the psychiatrist.

Another practical matter is that the examination I conduct may not be sufficient to make the decision about competency. I may need outside input. I may need to talk with other people who are relevant to the issue of competency. I need to have reliable sources, usually family members or the attorney. I need to see other data such as previous hospital records and medical records. Does the patient have fluctuating clarity or physical instability? What are the medical and psychological problems that accompany his decision making ability?

COMPETENCY OF THE ATTORNEY

When we speak of competency to stand trial, the major question is: "Does the defendant understand the nature and consequences of his legal situation"; i.e., does he know what he is involved in and what the consequences are? A person who is standing trial also has to be able to work with his attorney in preparing a rational defense. Sometimes after I examine a person and think he's competent, the lawyer calls and disagrees with me saying, "How can you say that? I can't get anything out of him. He's totally irrational with me." I may suggest a very concrete notion to use when observing the dyadic relationship between the defendant and his attorney. Sometimes this attorney is absolutely right. He's totally incompetent in the manner in which he asks the defendant questions. If the defendant is mentally retarded or has a severe psychosis and the lawyer has no patience, I may have to teach the lawyer how to ask the questions in order to make him competent with his client. The clinical skills we develop in psychiatry can easily be taught to attorneys in these instances just as attorneys have taught us a number of things about how we should approach certain clients they have with their particular problems.

CASE EXAMPLES

To illustrate the potential confusion in determining competency, let us take a couple of actual cases that have been decided in the courts. In the case of State v. Hayes, Mr. Hayes was found to have committed a crime or at least was charged with it in New Hampshire and was sent to prison. In prison it was decided that he should be in the hospital because he was found to be incompetent to stand trial. When he was in the hospital he was given medication and while on medication he became competent. He knew then that he was scheduled to stand trial for a serious crime and stopped his medication. He became incompetent to stand trial but was sent to court and tried anyway. On appeal the Supreme Court of New Hampshire upheld the decision by saying that there are two conflicting issues in terms of competency. One is the right to be tried as a competent person and the other is the right to refuse medication if one is competent to do so. The court said (and I paraphrase), "Mr. Hayes, when you were competent, you competently refused the medication, a right which you have and which the doctors upheld. But you did that knowing that this would render you incompetent to stand trial - you can't have it both ways; we are going to try you because you competently waived your right to be tried as a competent person."

The second case I want to raise is that of State v. Davee (1977) regarding who makes the decision and are they competent to decide? The case has to do with a man who was found not guilty by reason of insanity and was sent to the state hospital for treatment. While at the hospital, with treatment, he improved following an acute psychotic episode. He was no longer seen as mentally ill and no longer in need of hospitalization. In Missouri the judge decides when to release a patient to the street. Nobody can tell the judge that Davee is no longer dangerous, so the judge decided to keep him in the hospital. On appeal the Supreme Court of Missouri decided that even though the doctors had testified that Davee is no longer mentally ill and could not benefit from traditional hospital care, treatment was redefined to include observation and containment (preventive detention). I wonder whether that was a competent decision. It was certainly authoritative. The Davee decision has been nullified by subsequent case law.

The third case involves medicine and not specifically psychiatry. In this instance a 79 year old woman was wheeled into my office with a plastic bag over her foot. She was noted to have severe diabetes and gangrene of the leg for the past seven months. She had taken good care of her foot and the gangrene had not spread as she was told it would. She noted that her husband was marvelous at taking care of her. When I examined her she indicated that she was not going to have the operation on her foot and yet she knew that she would die if she did not have this operation. She was aware that she could get worse and become toxic, and that when she would become toxic she would be deemed incompetent and the foot would be taken off anyway. As we continued to talk I included her husband in the examination and she told me that she had taken care of him for ten years because of his heart condition and now it was her turn. She was receiving tremendous secondary gain having her husband take good care of her and paying great attention to her. At the end of the interview as she was leaving, she winked and told me, "You know doctor, I'm not going to let myself die; when the leg gets bad enough, I'll have it taken off, but I'm having such a good time now having my husband take care of me and my foot is not any worse." Naturally, I found this woman competent. The decision was made following the establishment of sufficient rapport to allow her to tell me what she wanted me to know.

It is important for the examining physician, whether he be a psychiatrist or not, to have a particular set of questions to ask a patient he is examining for competency. He should not have a set bias ahead of time, because the patient who appears to be incompetent, on close questioning, may in fact be quite competent to make decisions about her own medical treatment. The attitude, the manner in which the questions are asked, and the type of questions are all important in assessing a patient's competence to make decisions about his/her own treatment.

CONCLUSION

I will conclude this presentation with a brief summary of Norman Cousins' "The Anatomy of an Illness as Perceived by the Patient". Briefly noted, Norman Cousins, a former editor of the Saturday Review published this paper in the New England Journal of Medicine. He apparently developed a toxic blood disorder and was allowed by his doctor to help make decisions about the treatment of his illness when the usual medical regimen failed to bring improvement. The new treatment regimen suggested by Cousins seemed to work, he did improve and subsequently recovered. When he was out of danger he claimed that he was the luckiest patient alive - not because he had lived, but because he had a doctor who was willing to listent to him. From this beautiful story two caveats emerge regarding competency: 1. Doctors should listen to their patients. 2. To the extent possible, the patient should participate in the decision making about his own treatment.

REFERENCES

Wyatt v. Stickney, 325 F Supp. 781 MD, Ala. 1971.
Rouse v. Cameron, 373 F 2d, 451 DC Cir. 1966.
Donaldson v. O'Connor 493 F 2d, 507, 520 5th Cir. 1974.
Rogers v. Okin, 478 F Supp. (D. Mass. 1979).
Rennie v. Klein, 462 F Supp. 1131, 1145 (1978).
State v. Hayes, 389 A 2d, 1379.
State v. Davee, 558 SW 2d, 335 (1977).
Cousins, N (1976). The anatomy of an illness (as perceived by the patient). N Eng J Med 295, 26:1458.

Troubling Problems in Medical Ethics: The Third
Volume in a Series on Ethics, Humanism, and Medicine: 177–178
© 1981 Alan R. Liss, Inc., 150 Fifth Ave., New York, NY 10011

DISCUSSION SUMMARY: COMPETENCE AND THE RIGHT TO REFUSE
                      TREATMENT

Marc D. Basson
Director, CEHM
University of Michigan
Ann Arbor, Michigan

Virtually all the participants believed that the
patient described was competent to refuse treatment at the
beginning of the case and that he should have been sent home
at that time. They pointed out that Millburn's basic goals
(to survive and to alleviate his symptoms) seemed essentially
reasonable and that his disorientation to time did not render
him unable to process medical information. "If Millburn had
agreed to the operations, no one would have doubted his competence to consent, " pointed out one medical student. Another discussant added, "The fact that the doctors asked
Millburn to consent to these procedures means that they
believed him competent to give such consent. The mere fact
that he refuses their advice should not then be an excuse
for declaring him incompetent." The general consensus was
that Millburn's refusal should have been honored and he
should have been discharged as soon as it was clear that
he was adamant and not simply reacting to a misunderstanding
or to an abrupt physician. One group felt that they could
not be certain that Millburn's refusal was not born of reversible hospital-acquired disorientation and therefore
suggested that the surgeons speak to Millburn again in his
home weeks later with his family present and try to obtain
consent in this more familiar setting.

A few participants argued that Millburn had been incompetent from the beginning and that the surgeons should
have proceeded on the basis of Millburn's daughter's proxy
consent. These participants pointed to Millburn's disorientation, his questionable mental status exam, and his
refusal of further mental status testing. They agreed that

Millburn's aims of preserving his life and alleviating his symptoms were reasonable 'and claimed that the physicians should do their best to achieve these goals for Millburn (by operating) rather than allowing themselves to be dissuaded by Millburn's irrational fears and inability to comprehend the unlikelihood of his death from the proposed operations.

Those who believed Millburn to be initially competent were prepared to retract this judgment as the case progressed and Millburn's mental status deteriorated. There was little question in anyone's mind that Millburn was incompetent as the case closed. Nevertheless, few participants were willing at that point to operate based on the daughter's proxy consent. One nurse summed up most of her group's feelings when she said, "The hospital has made Mr. Millburn sick and confused. This does not give them the right to take advantage of his confusion." Most participants felt that Millburn's previous and competent refusal of treatment ought to be considered controlling. A lawyer in one discussion group reminded discussants that physicians are supposed to have a fiduciary relationship with their patients and further argued that for Millburn's physicians to take advantage of Millburn's temporary incompetence to operate would constitute a serious breach of trust.

**Troubling Problems in Medical Ethics: The Third
Volume in a Series on Ethics, Humanism, and Medicine: 179–182
© 1981 Alan R. Liss, Inc., 150 Fifth Ave., New York, NY 10011**

INTRODUCTION: WHEN DOCTOR AND NURSE DISAGREE

Daria Chapelsky
CEHM
University of Michigan
Ann Arbor, Michigan

A certain amount of conflict is inherent in the physician-nurse relationship, not only between the physician and nurse but also between moral principles deriving from the organization of the hospital and those deriving from moral intuitions of the participants. A moral dilemma may arise in which the nurse must evaluate her own principles and weigh them against institutional demands for obedience. Two major sources of such conflict involve incompatibilities in professional roles and disagreements over moral judgments.

First, conflicts emerge from different professional roles involving different personal and professional obligations and loyalties. The physician's role is to alleviate the pain and suffering of the sick; his only loyalty is to the patient. The nurse's role is both patient advocacy and assistance to the physician and administration, and thus conflict is born. She is obligated to adhere to the American Nursing Association Code for Nurses which requires her to act as she believes right, to protect her clients, and to be fully accountable for her professional behavior (Aroskar, Flaherty, and Smith, 1977). Yet, her contract also charges her with professional obligations to uphold the (utilitarian) goals of the administrators of the health care institution and to obey the doctors they have hired. The greatest conflict in the nursing profession involves professional autonomy versus rigid institutional authoritarianism. Yet the nurse must recognise that sometimes she may be wrong and the institution right. To what extent ought the nurse engage in moral reasoning based on her personal moral values rather than those dictated by her institution?

A second source of conflict is evident in the manner in which each professional makes decisions and the extent to which he is able to act on his decisions. The physician is central to decision making in most hospitals while the nurse is relegated to following orders within the physician's framework. Authoritarian control over decision making may often be accompanied by similar dominance of the institution's communication system. According to Catherine Murphy, "the network of communication in the hospital hierarchy allows the physician to move freely throughout the institution, while the nurse communicates through proper bureaucratic channels." (Murphy, 1978). Stein has described the elaborate ploys to which nurses must often resort for communication with physicians in his paper "The Doctor-Nurse Game." (Stein, 1967).

In the case presented for discussion, an ethical dilemma is created by personal and situational conflicts between physician and nurse. The physician is instituting continuous supportive care for a dying patient. The nurse believes that this treatment should be discontinued to relieve the family's suffering and avoid prolonging the patient's life unduly. The nurse is therefore uncomfortable with carrying out the physician's orders and must decide what to do. Her role-specific obligations impel her toward obedience while personal and professional obligations toward patient and family seem to push her in the opposite direction. Should she comply, quit, or approach the family with her point of view? If she chooses the last of these, how will this influence her future interactions with physicians and the relationship of the physician with this patient and her family?

Our two speakers are well acquainted with this sort of ethical dilemma and both agree that conflict between physician and nurse ought to be resolved through appropriate communication. Upon closer reading, however, we see that they differ distinctly in what they believe constitutes appropriate and effective communication.

Dr. Bartlett suggests that when a disagreement evolves because of differing judgments, whether medical or moral, the nurse should initiate direct communication with the physician, requesting clarification. Once the nurse has raised an issue, it then becomes the physician's responsibility to explain his view. Bartlett hopes that such explanation will usually resolve the problem, but suggests that if it does not the nurse may explain her own perceptions or even appeal to a supervisory physician if one exists. Bartlett claims that such a process will amicably resolve virtually all doctor-nurse disagreements. For the remaining few, Bartlett simply points out that someone must always make final decisions and that within the hospital setting the physician is the captain of the team, the ultimate authority on patient care.

Dr. Aroskar interprets disagreement between physician and nurse as occuring at the interface between politics and ethics. The nurse's position in the hospital hierarchy and the various claims on her loyalty and accountability are intricately bound up in her ethical crisis. Aroskar considers the hospital setting "deterrent to professional nursing," increasing communication problems and the risks to nurses if they behave ethically. She stresses that it is not so easy for a nurse either to open communication or to use it satis-factorily within the authoritarian hospital hierarchy. In the best of all possible worlds, Aroskar would have nurse and physician cooperating as professionals of equal status, rather than having the physician dictate orders to the nurse.

While both speakers want doctors and nurses to communi-cate, they differ on the intent and form of such communica-tion. Aroskar would like to see communication begin before decisions are made that need to be challenged. She envisions a decision making process in which "everyone's goals and values would be taken into consideration" at the outset. Bartlett, on the other hand, reminds us that every team must have a captain. "Communication has to start with the nurse," he writes, "because the disagreement starts with the nurse." While he rejects blatant authoritarianism and insists that physicians need to listen to other health care personnel, Bartlett nevertheless believes that so long as the physician takes care of the patient he must make the ultimate decisions. If the patient does not like them, Bartlett reminds us, he always has the option of changing physicians, but when the patient chooses to continue his current doctor-patient relationship, other health care personnel should be wary of interfering with it.

REFERENCES

Aroskar MA, Flaherty MJ, Smith JM (1977). The nurse and
    orders not to resuscitate. Hastings Center Report
    7(4):27.
Jameton A (1977). The nurse: When roles and rules conflict.
    Hastings Center Report 7(4):22.
Murphy CP (1978). The moral situation in nursing. In
    Bandman EL, Bandman B (eds)(1978). "Bioethics and
    Human Rights: A Reader for Health Professionals."
    Boston: Little, Brown and Company.
Stein LI (1967). The doctor-nurse game. Arch Gen Psychiat
    16:699.

**Troubling Problems in Medical Ethics: The Third
Volume in a Series on Ethics, Humanism, and Medicine: 183–185
© 1981 Alan R. Liss, Inc., 150 Fifth Ave., New York, NY 10011**

WHEN DOCTOR AND NURSE DISAGREE

CASE FOR DISCUSSION

Ann Schneider was a 27 year old woman who had been admitted to the hospital with fulminant hepatitis (inflammation of the liver) and progressive cirrhosis. Despite elaborate diagnostic and therapeutic efforts, her physicians were unable to arrest or even clearly explain her disease. Her kidneys failed as well and she was diagnosed as having hepatorenal syndrome, in which the patient's liver and kidneys fail and death almost invariably results. As her disease worsened, she became comatose.

After several days, Mr. Schneider approaches Dr. Manning (the chief resident) and asks whether Mrs. Schneider might ever recover. "If not," he asks, "shouldn't I make some decisions or something? Ann wouldn't want to be kept this way unless there was a chance."

Dr. Manning replied that Mrs. Schneider's condition was indeed critical but that he did not believe he or any other doctor could ever say with absolute certainty that a disease process was irreversible. "We can't give up," he says. "People sometimes wake up even when we're sure they won't. Every day we keep her alive is another day a miracle might happen and she might get better." Mr. Schneider agrees to let Dr. Manning continue aggressive therapy.

Elizabeth Cornwall has been head nurse in the intensive care unit for six years and has been an ICU nurse for the last seventeen. She is disturbed by the aggressive nature of Dr. Manning's therapeutic plan. She has seen many patients comatose with hepatorenal syndrome. None have survived.

She looks up the syndrome in the hospital library and finds
no cases reported in which a patient with hepatorenal syndrome
as severe as Mrs. Schneider's has recovered.

She complains to Dr. Manning that she and her nurses do
not understand why Mrs. Schneider is being treated in this
way. She describes the current call orders and therapeutic
plan as illogical and impossible for her to carry out in
good faith. "This woman is dying," she says, "if not already
dead for all practical purposes. We nurses are much closer
to the patient than you are. We're with them all the time
and we can tell when someone is hopeless. I've read about
this disease. People like her just don't wake up. I wouldn't
feel right trying to resuscitate her if she arrests, either.
It just doesn't make sense to keep wasting time, money, and
effort on her, not to mention what we're putting her poor
husband through."

Manning agrees that his knowledge of hepatorenal syndrome
coincides with hers. "You're right," he says, "no one like
this has ever woken up. But if we don't try, how will we
know?"

"You give up," he continued, "when you can't get any
blood into a vein. As long as she's breathing and her
heart's beating, tend to her. You can't know what will
happen. When a doctor says a patient is beyond help, he's
really admitting his lack of willingness to fight. Some say
we prolong life too often. But the people whose lives are
prolonged don't say that. It's always the healthy survivors
who insist on the patient's right to die with dignity."*

"It's my job to decide how the patient ought to be
treated and your's to carry it out," Dr. Manning concludes.
He turns and walks away.

Ms. Cornwall tries to discuss her problem with the
hospital's director of nursing, but is told that only physicians
have the power to dictate therapy. The director suggests
she try talking with Dr. Manning again, but Ms. Cornwall
knows that this would be useless. The director also warns
her against allowing the family to sense her misgivings

———————

*quoted from Emil J. Freireich, MD in Ross (1972). See
references at end of volume.

about the therapy since this would interfere with their confidence in the doctor and the hospital.

The point here is not whether Ms. Cornwall is right and Dr. Manning is wrong. Instead, consider the following. Ms. Cornwall believes that Mrs. Schneider's condition is hopeless and that if Mr. Schneider knew this he would want her placed on "do not resuscitate" status. She believes that Mr. Schneider is being misled by Dr. Manning. Yet she also recognizes that Manning is a physician and that he has more medical training than she. Given that she believes these things, what ought she to do? Does she have an obligation to the patient or the patient's family to ensure that they are fully informed and appropriately treated? Should this supersede her contractual obligations to obey the orders of the director of nursing and of Dr. Manning? Should she talk to Mr. Schneider directly? Allow him to "sense her misgivings about the treatment" and hope that he will ask her about them? Should she withdraw from the case? Is the disagreement here medical or moral?

(Case prepared by Daria Chapelsky and Marc D. Basson.)

**Troubling Problems in Medical Ethics: The Third
Volume in a Series on Ethics, Humanism, and Medicine: 187-192**
© **1981 Alan R. Liss, Inc., 150 Fifth Ave., New York, NY 10011**

WHEN DOCTOR AND NURSE DISAGREE: AN INTERFACE OF POLITICS
AND ETHICS

Mila Ann Aroskar, R.N., Ed.D.

School of Public Health
University of Minnesota
Minneapolis, Minnesota

One interpretive statement in the ANA Code for Nurses
with Interpretive Statements (1976) states: "The interde-
pendent relationship of the nursing and medical professions
requires collaboration around the need of the client and
among other requirements, deliberations in determining functional relationships of medicine and nursing". We need
clarification and illumination of these relationships which
cannot be done in professional isolation.

The nurse's social position in most bureaucratice organizations and the potential problem of multiple sources of
loyalty and accountability underlie many of the ethical
problems faced by nurses. Some examples of multiple sources
of loyalty and accountability include: feelings of loyalty
and accountability to the patient/client, to the physician
or physicians, to one's self, to the employing institution,
to the nursing profession, and to the state as most states
have nurse practice acts.

What is it like to be a nurse in an intensive care unit?
This is a question with ethical dimensions in the sense that
ethical inquiry has as one aspect the identification of the
context of ethical issues and dilemmas. One nurse who left
ICU nursing told the author, "The doctor comes in and briefly looks at the patients, writes order, and leaves. As a
nurse, I was obligated to care for patients in this ethically laden situation without benefit of any discussion or
input into decisions affecting nursing care of patients and
use of nursing resources. I found this to be the most difficult aspect of caring for patients in an ICU". One unresolved issue is who should make and have input into decisions

where the ethical dimensions and concerns predominate.
Many professional and lay people still consider the physician
to be the "captain of the ship". Yet, the burden of decisions made by others frequently falls on nurses as revealed
in the previous quotation. Similar remarks have been made
to me on numerous occasions by nurses who work in intensive
care settings which are areas of great psychological and
emotional stress.

Research findings provide clues to the ICU environment
which many nurses experience. Some of these are: repetitive
exposure to death and dying, an overshelming work load, too
much responsibility, poor communication between nurses and
physicians, and limited work space. Other aspects of the
larger social context for ICU nurses include the highly
stratified bureaucratic institution in which they practice
(Davis, 1979). The social system of the hospital has been
discussed as a deterrent to professional nursing. The following characteristics of hospitals do act as deterrents to
professional nursing: frequent downward communication of
orders, rules and proscribed procedures issued by persons in
authority, inadequate channels for upward communication of
plans, suggestions and complaints originating on the lower
hierarchical levels of nursing, limited lateral communication,
and psychologic isolation.

The above characteristics and other variables such as
the paternalism of many physicians and the characteristics
of nurses themselves such as obedience to authority have
lead some authors to raise questions regarding to what extent nurses in such institutions can be ethical. And if
they to practice ethically, what is the potential price they
may have to pay for their actions? Does one have to be a
hero or heroine in order to be ethical? Incidentally, I
have found in talking with medical students that many of them
are faced with questions similar to those faced by nurses
who seek to practice in an ethical manner, for example,
whistle blowing.

To pay attention to ethical dimensions of situations in
ICUs and other settings, one should consider the following
in a systematic way: 1. what the nurse, physician, patient,
family member, etc. should or ought to do in a situation
where there is conflict or confrontation between individual
human needs and the welfare of others; 2. there is a choice
to be made between alternatives which often seem equally
unattractive, remembering that a choice to do nothing also

has consequences; 3. consideration of moral principles such
as doing no harm, keeping a promise, assuring autonomy in
looking at alternatives for action; and 4. consider that
choices are affected by feelings of the individuals involved
which are frequently caused by the situation and the context
of the situation such as an ICU setting.

Interface the above ethical dimensions with some dimensions of the political realm. Concepts of politics include:
politics as the art of the possible; the art of adjusting and
ordering interacting and conflicting relationships between
individuals and groups; competition for control, power, and
leadership between competing interest groups or individuals;
and politics as public or social ethics, that is, discerning
the morally preferable from among practical possibilities,
or clarifying the relevant moral principles.

One begins to discern some of the broader aspects of the
situation which a disagreement between a doctor and nurse
or medicine and nursing represents as each struggles with
what is identified as an ethical dilemma in an ICU setting.
The situation involves not only individuals but groups within the institution and the larger community. Different
levels of the health care system will affect and be affected
by efforts to resolve such situations for the benefit of
the patient/client whether it is the individual, group or
family, or the community.

I would like to talk briefly about four different views
of health care that can be used as models in thinking about
the questions we have before us at this conference. If
nurses, patients/clients and other providers hold incongru-
ent views of the health care system, this will affect if and
how disagreements are defined and resolved in the ethical
and other realms. This discussion is based on the views
described by Newton, a philosopher, in an article on the
accountability of the nurse (1979). These views will probably sound familiar to you. The first view is "health care
as a commodity". In this view, medicine, health care or
health are commodities offered for sale by institutions
called hospitals or clinics. The patient is a consumer;
the physician is an outside contractor; and nurses are
viewed as employees. Kindness to patients and deference to
physicians on the part of nurses are considered to be praiseworthy characteristics, but an employee's responsibility is
to the immediate superior in the institutional organization.
Institutional interests take precedence over the competing

interests of traditional professional medical privileges or patient/client needs. On this view, one could argue that the nurse in a disagreement with a physician should follow the direction of her superior in the nursing hierarchy under some principle of obedience to a higher authority or decide disagreements on the basis of institutional interests. Generally, this would be a more utilitarian approach. These actions seem to negate principles of self-determination and respect for the individual - directly for the nurse and indirectly for the client/patient. It may enhance to some degree these principles for the physician.

The second view is "health care as medical cases or scientific projects". In this view of health care as simply a series of projects with the cure of diseases as the object, then the physician could be viewed as the scientist who carries on the project or experiment. The hospital is the laboratory and the patient is the subject matter. Nurses and other health professionals carry on small projects as part of the physicians' projects. Nurses are accountable only to the physician for each case or project. The hospital and its employees exist only to assist all the projects within its walls. Patients contribute nothing because they don't have the required knowledge to participate, a passive role. This view is somewhat analagous to the concept of the hospital as the doctor's workshop. Again, this view enhances the autonomy of the individual physician, but negates the principle for others involved. One could also ask whether or not the principle of telling the truth is enhanced or negated in a situation as described in our case study. The family apparently does not have all the available information to make a knowledgeable decision. This is ethically questionable. One might also ask about the harm which accrues to all the individuals involved, including the physician, who are struggling with their decisions. These two models of health care as a commodity and as scientific projects imply the possibility of various degrees of coercion of employees, patients and families which decreases their freedom in making choices.

The third view is "health care as implementation of a right to relief from pain". The focus of health care is seen as the patient's right to relief from a painful or debilitating condition in this view. The hospital is seen as society's instrument for the implementation of that right. The nurse's first responsibility is to the patient, his needs and wants. The idea of care based on patient need is more

characteristic of the ANA Code. At this time, it may be difficult for nurses to put patient interests before hospital
interests due at least partly to characteristics of bureaucratic organizations, but the trend is in favor of the patient.
Consider the AHA Patient Bill of Rights, consumer activities
in health, and expanding areas of health law. Under this
model, the patient/client may be in a position to terrify
employed providers with the prospect of a malpractice suit.
This could be more of a threat than the prospect of getting
fired. As you recall, we asked the question early on as to
whether or not someone has to be a hero or heroine in order
to be ethical. On this view, the patient has the right to
control not only the means of the relief of his or her complaint but also how it is defined. In such a situation,
the nurse, patient and physician may well disagree. Only
the patient can evaluate when the pain is gone or the condition relieved or improved. Providers would in effect be
answerable to the patient/client. The patient's standards
would be paramount in decision-making.

The fourth view is "health care as promotion of well-
being" or what I like to think of as the cooperative community view. If health care is seen as promoting the well-being
of persons, as opposed to curing disease or catering to
wants, then each profession may become more autonomous in
that the patient/client, physicians, nurses, and other providers will focus on the enterprise of furthering that individual's well-being. Disagreements between physicians
and nurses, in this view, would focus on decision-making
which enhances patient/client well-being. The values of
all involved would be part of the decision-making process
at least in terms of identifying those values and goals.
The patient/client is expected to set aside counterproductive
wants and demands to participate in his or her own recovery
and care. In this view, each person becomes accountable for
his own performance or activities in relation to the well-
being of a particular individual, group or community. For
example, the nurse would become more accountable to professional standards and carrying out a process of ethical inquiry in situations where professional and ethical dimensions
were predominant before making decisions.

The fourth view is the view of health care which I find
more desireable than the other three in terms of promoting
the autonomy of all involved, at least theoretically. Everyone's goals and values would be taken into consideration as

part of the decision-making process. This view also enhances and expresses the principle of respect for all the individuals involved. The predominating view held in an institution whether it is the health care as a commodity view, implementation of a right to relief from pain view, scientific projects view, or promotion of well-being view could dictate the "ethics" of the institution and how disagreements between physicians and nurses can and should be resolved. However, as we all know, individuals hold single or multiple views of health and health care which may well conflict in any given situation. However, determining views of those in a situation could be another piece of data needed for clarification and critical systematic reflection <u>before</u> making decisions which involve the ethical and political realms. One is attempting to order conflicting relationships when there are unequal power ratios and bring ethical principles to bear on a specific situation.

I have not touched on the ethical principle of distributive justice due to time limitations but suggest that this is a significant issue in the case study. I hope that our discussion of the issues raised by the case study will proceed in a spirit of compassion toward everyone involved. As providers, we are all present or potential patients/clients in the health care community where polities and ethics do interface. Thank you.

REFERENCES

Davis AJ (March 1979). Ethics Rounds with Intensive Care
   Nurses. Nursing Clinics of North America 14:48-50.
Newton L (October 1979). To Whom is the Nurse Accountable?
   A Philosophical Perspective. Connecticut Medicine 43:7-9.

Troubling Problems in Medical Ethics: The Third
Volume in a Series on Ethics, Humanism, and Medicine: 193–202
© 1981 Alan R. Liss, Inc., 150 Fifth Ave., New York, NY 10011

WHEN DOCTOR AND NURSE DISAGREE

Robert H. Bartlett, M.D.

University of Michigan Department of Surgery

Box 056, Ann Arbor, Michigan

Dr. Aroskar stated this problem so nicely, and laid out
the principles so clearly that I really don't have a great
deal to add. Unfortunately for the discussion, I don't have
great disagreement with what she said, so we can't have a
flaming argument.

Let me reduce the case example to an issue, and propose
an immediate solution. We have a sick patient, under the
care of a doctor, and another informed person thinks the
care is incorrect. The other informed person could be
another doctor, or a physical therapist, or a consultant, or
a nurse, anyone. That's the problem. In the circumstance
we are to discuss today the informed person is responsible
for carrying out the directions of the doctor who is in
charge. That relationship might exist between an intern and
a resident, a resident and a consultant, a nurse and a physician, a LPN and an RN; whoever it is, there is someone who
is in charge, and there is someone who disagrees with what
is going on, but is charged with carrying out that particular aspect of care. The solution to the problem as Mila has
already pointed out, is to sit down and talk about it, discuss it. Communication virtually always resolves the problem. The only thing I would add is, it is important to
resolve the problem in a way that does not interfere with
what you might call the doctor/patient relationship, or the
interplay between the physician who is in charge and the
patient and the patient's family. Those of you who do not
work in this milieu every day should know that disagreement
is exceedingly uncommon in relation to the total number of
medical care transactions. The vast majority of patients,

doctors, and nurses work together very smoothly. So when a disagreement occurs, it is an unusual circumstance; hence we tend to focus on it.

There are three categories of disagreement. The first is a simple lack of communication. The second is a scientific disagreement over what is or is not the correct way to proceed. The third, and the thorniest, is a philosophical or ethical disagreement over a value system. A communication problem can be resolved, or at least clarified, by simple discussion. It does require the ability and the willingness to talk about the disagreement, which requires an action on the part of both parties. The scientific category is one in which the doctor has embarked on a course of action and the nurse thinks he knows a better way. (Please indulge me if I assign a gender to personal pronouns). The third, the philosophical or ethical disagreement, simply boils down to discussion of value systems. The discussion is, "We have made different value judgments; we should pursue what I think is the correct set of values in behalf of this patient." Of course, these categories might overlap, but usually a problem can be reduced to one of these three.

Since the majority of the audience here are students who have not yet become directly involved in these inter-relationships (except, perhaps, as the patient) we should define the background for potential disagreement.

First someone gets sick. He contacts a doctor saying, in essence, "Will you care for me?" The doctor makes a decision. She may say, "No, I don't do that"; or, "I suggest you find another doctor"; that is her prerogative. But as soon as the doctor says, "Take two aspirin and call me in the morning", she has initiated a contract. She is committed to undertake the care of the patient for the duration of the illness, perhaps for a lifetime. The patient and the patient's family may break the agreement at any time. Anywhere along the line they can say, "I think you are not doing the right thing. I would like someone else to do it." The patient very rarely does, however, because of a normal human desire to believe that the doctor is doing her best in any situation. The patient proceeds on that assumption, and that is a fair assumption. The doctor is obligated, morally, legally, ethically, and for every other reason, to do what she feels is best for the patient. That doesn't necessarily mean all that is absolutely medically

possible for the patient; sometimes the best treatment is
not the maximum treatment.

That trust which is shared between the doctor and the
patient is, in fact, the doctor/patient relationship. It
is a first principle when considering disagreements over
care. Even the cynical pessimist who takes it upon himself
to generalize that doctors are money-grubbing people who
don't care about patients, or that nurses are lazy and presumptuous, even such a pessimist will usually say, "But my
doctor is a dedicated physician, or my nurse is a compassionate person."

This relationship lasts over a long time, in and out
of the hospital, and is important to keep in mind when we
get down to discussing specific facts. To disrupt that
trust has far-reaching psychological implications on the
patient and the family which may interfere with recovery
from the disease process. A person who disagrees with the
course of treatment must consider all the negative and positive factors of intervening before approaching the patient
or family.

The hospital-based nurse and other paramedical people
get involved in that relationship when the patient is admitted to the hospital. Although a professional dedicated
nurse (or physical therapist, or resident, or whoever) is
absolutely committed to the best in scientific and humanistic
care of the patient, that person's responsibility is essentially to carry out the job as defined by the hospital and
by the physician who is directing the care. His contract
lasts for the duration of the time clock. When the shift
is over, he can go home. If he doesn't like what is going
on, he can take a different patient the next day. He
doesn't carry a beeper. He doesn't follow the patient over
months or years. He doesn't get calls from the patient's
relatives or lawyer or insurance company. He has a different level of commitment.

Now those are the cold hard facts, but those of you
who are nurses or physical therapists may well say, "Don't
tell me that, fella, I care. I take my patients home. I
spend more time with them than the doctor. I stick with
them until they live or die." Of course you do. That is
the mark of a professional. In practice, nurses develop in-
credible loyalty to their nursing unit, to patient care, to

patients personally, and to the families of the patients
personally. This is especially true in critical care units,
where the emotional intensity is high and the care is highly
specialized. The nurse derives a great sense of satisfaction
from combining expert science and compassionate care. In
practice, the wise doctor recognizes that and views care of
the patient as a team effort. By inviting discussion, the
doctor encourages everyone to act as a professional in
caring for the patient. Nonetheless, the doctor is "where
the buck stops". She makes the decision in an authoritarian
democracy. We don't decide on treatment by a show of hands -
there is one person who has to call the shots. The patient
and the family have their relationship with that one person,
so you can see how it comes full cycle.

That's a long-winded explanation of the background, but
if you don't work in this field every day, it is important
that you understand it. Some nurses and other health care
professionals would not like my description of the background. It might be called paternalistic, or onesided, or
insensitive. If doctors abuse the system and ignore their
counterpart professionals, those adjectives do apply. But,
like it or not, that is the system under which we currently
operate.

Now, the topic is, what happens when a doctor and nurse
disagree? With that background in mind, what "disagree"
means is that the doctor has embarked on a course of treatment and the nurse thinks that he knows a better course of
treatment. In other words, the nurse reacts to what the
doctor has done. Therefore, "disagreements" are always on
the part of the person who is not initiating the treatment.
The doctor has written the orders; she doesn't disagree
with what she has written. She has done the best she can
for the patient. So, given that little bit of redefinition
of what disagreement means, let us talk about the three
categories.

Poor communication, as I have said, is far and away the
most common problem. One classic definition comes from the
movie, Cool Hand Luke, in which Paul Newman plays the prisoner and the stubby red-necked warden of a little Southern
jail says, "What we have heah is a failure to communicate."
What the warden means is, "I say what to do and you do it.
If you don't do it, that is a failure to communicate."
This should never happen in medical practice, but it does.

The physician's responsibility is to never be in the position of the warden who considers communication a strict one-
way directive. The communication we are talking about has
to start with the nurse, because the disagreement starts
with the nurse. If the nurse doesn't say, "Why are we doing this?", the communication never begins. The doctor may
not spontaneously say, "Today we are doing this because of
that." Usually she will walk in, review the patient's condition, write a set of orders and say, "Here are the orders.
I'll be back in six hours. Tell me if anything happens."
She won't initiate a dialogue unless the person who disagrees asks, "Why are the orders the way they are?" Usually
any disagreement will be resolved by just talking about it.

The second category is scientific or medical disagreement. It arises when the nurse thinks he knows (or does
know) more than the doctor in a given circumstance. This
occurs in highly specialized intensive care units. In a
burn unit, or a neonatal intensive care unit, or an emergency room, for example, a nurse or a resident may know
much more about what is going on than any particular physician who happens to have a patient in that unit at that time.
Such disagreements are rarely problems, because somewhere
up the line there is a physician director of that unit or
that particular activity who knows at least as much as the
nurse knows, and they can agree on a procedure or protocol.
The prophylaxis for scientific disagreement, then, is previously prepared protocols. If serious disagreements still
arise, the first step is communication. The nurse should
ask the prescribing physician why she is doing what she is
doing. The insecure physician might react negatively to
such a question. If so, perhaps the suggestion would be
better directed to the physician who is in charge of the
unit. The second step, then, is going to the physician who
is ultimately in charge of the case (if the disagreement is
with a resident, as in the case example) and/or to the
physician in charge of the unit, and moving the scientific
discussion to that level. The solution to a scientific
dilemma is not, certainly, to go to the family or the patient.
They have a relationship established with the doctor. To
say to them, "You know, your doctor has prescribed this,
but it really would be much better to do this, from a scientific point of view", obviously is going to disrupt that
relationship, and may have much more devastating effects
than any particular choice in treatment.

For example, suppose a lady has breast cancer. She and her family and her surgeon discuss treatment. After considering the alternatives, the patient decides on the treatment her surgeon recommends, let us say, a partial mastectomy and axillary node dissection. The patient is admitted to the hospital and some well-meaning person says, "You know, the results are better with a radical mastectomy"; or "Local radiation is just as good but less disabling"; or "Don't have a node dissection, it doesn't improve your chances." All these statements are scientifically correct, but to present such opinions directly to the patient is simply meddling with the patient's psychological well-being. It is appropriate for a concerned nurse (or radiation therapist or social worker) to ask the surgeon why she and the patient decided on a particular course of treatment, if the question is motivated by a desire to help the patient cope with her disease.

The last category is philosophical disagreement, and this is the most difficult. When I started medical school here many years ago, the dean was a wise and perceptive man named William Hubbard. When we assembled on the first day of medical school, Hubbard said, "Gentlemen" (there were actually a few ladies in the class, but he referred to the class as gentlemen) "the practice of medicine is 99 percent grandmother and one percent science. So much for the grandmother, we will now spend four years on the science." He was right. You must spend time learning the science, but 99 percent of the practice is, indeed, grandmother. Grandma was usually right in value judgements. She could point out the pros and cons, and suggest the best thing to do. When we are talking about philosophical or ethical dilemmas we are talking about value judgements. Someone says, "I have a value judgment and you have a different value judgment. Which is correct?" The tendency is to say, "Mine is correct, because I believe it." Reduced to the terms of an individual patient, weighty dilemmas arise.

For example, suppose a patient has metastatic colon cancer. The doctor and the patient and the family talk about chemotherapy. Chemotherapy might extend the patient's life for a few months. It doesn't have any effect on ultimate survival. It has unpleasant side effects. The doctor asks, "What would you like to do?" The patient always says, "What would you suggest?" He doesn't want to make the choice, nor should he have to. He has not seen 80, or 100,

or 600 people who have colon cancer and what happens to
them, nor has he seen 600 people who have had chemotherapy
and its complications, so he must rely on the doctor's
judgment. The doctor knows that she can relate what she
would suggest, what she would do for herself, and she also
knows that the patient will grasp for any hope. Generally
speaking the patient and family will say, "If there is
something to do let's do it." Laetril, herbs, wishful
thinking, Cytoxan, all fit into the same category in that
particular disease. If the doctor says to the patient,
"I think you ought to just go home or take a trip to Europe
and forget the chemotherapy", that is very honest and very
sincere advice but it may not answer the patient's quest for
support. The patient will probably find another doctor who
says, "I think we ought to give you a full course of chemotherapy. It costs 60 dollars a day but it might prolong
your life."

I paint that background, and ask you to imagine what
might happen three months later if the patient has elected
chemotherapy and has developed complications. He has a
low white count, pneumonia, is bleeding from every orifice
and feels miserable. He comes into the hospital, where the
nurse enters the scene. The nurse may say, "This is tor-
ture. What are we doing this for?" What the nurse is
really saying is, "I've made a judgment about the quality
of life. I judge that this patient's quality of life isn't
as good as I would like to see it, therefore, why don't
you stop what you are doing?" On the other hand, suppose
the patient did not elect chemotherapy, and comes into the
hospital three months later with metastatic cancer in the
lung, jaundice, bleeding from every orifice, and miserable.
A nurse might say, "Why isn't this patient on chemotherapy?
What is going on here? I've seen patients on chemotherapy
and they do fine. I've made a judgment about this person's
quality of life and I feel it would be better if you put
him on chemotherapy. I have a big disagreement."

Now I point out those situations as examples of philosophical value judgment dilemmas, which the people involved may perceive as scientific dilemmas. Although the
nurse says, "There has been a scientific decision here regarding chemotherapy and I disagree with it", it is actually
a value judgment; a discussion about the quality of life or
the longevity of life.

The case example falls into this category. The nurse is saying that her opinion regarding the patient's quality of life should take precedence. She presumes that the husband has not been fully informed and if he were he would favor withdrawing treatment. It is a common but presumptuous condition of mankind--to assume that our own value system is more correct than others simply because we believe in it.

The prophylaxis for this kind of dilemma is discussion, group meetings, getting together the physicians, nurses, therapists, residents and families involved. If we embark on a course, and everybody knows the rationale, then there is less likelihood of arriving at philosophical dilemmas.

When the situation does arise, again, I would advise the person who disagrees with what is being done to ask the physician first. If that does not solve the disagreement, go to the physician who is ultimately in charge of that particular discipline or arrange a group meeting. If the dilemma persists, and you think your opinion must be stated to the family, the way to do it is to be sure that the family knows that they can opt for another physician. Now, the patient and family should know that from day one. They have been given a description of the "patient's bill of rights" on admission to the hospital. They have been told that they may refuse care or change physicians, but they forget it because of the doctor/patient relationship. Most patients don't want to think, "Maybe this doctor is not doing it right, and anytime I want to I can shift to someone else." They think, "This person is doing the best she can for myself, or my wife, or whomever it happens to be." Occasionally, it is useful to remind the family that they can select any physician or hospital they wish, but consider all the consequences first.

As an aside, that was the bottom line in the Karen Ann Quinlan case. The newspaper reporting of that particular ethical dilemma was quite misleading. The actual opinion of the judge was very wise. Remember, the discussion was that the family wanted a comatose girl taken off the ventilator, and the doctor wouldn't do it. (It was only an academic courtroom exercise because the girl didn't need to be on the ventilator anyway.) The headlines read "Court says girl must stay on ventilator." But what the judge actually said was, in essence, "This is not for me to decide. This is a medical decision. It isn't a legal decision. If you don't

like the doctor's advice, get another doctor." Pretty good.
He also said, "This has become such an inflammatory issue
that I'm going to appoint a separate legal guardian to advise you all on how to proceed." The legal guardian said,
"Get another doctor," which they did.

The final solution for the professional who has a value
judgment disagreement is to withdraw. In the case example
the nurse is urging termination of treatment because she
thinks the patient and her husband would prefer it. Her
unstated frustration is, "This circumstance is emotionally
uncomfortable for me and my staff and we have to be at the
bedside eight hours at a time." Everyone in medicine experiences this feeling, and a decision to be excused from
a case should always be honored. In this case withdrawing
is the best solution and will not change the ultimate outcome. If the nurse were urging more vigorous treatment
(with dialysis, or a liver transplant, for example) which
might alter the outcome, the disagreement becomes a scientific one, for which a scientific answer could be provided.

Summary: In the doctor/patient relationship, the doctor is obligated to explain the alternatives and provide the
best care for the patient. The patient and his family are
entitled to the trust that the doctor will provide the best
care. Another health care professional who proposes that
another method of treatment is better should first check his
premises, and, second, consider al the implications of
making such a proposal to the patient or family.

When doctor and nurse "disagree", it is the nurse who
disagrees with the course of treatment which the doctor and
patient have planned. If the disagreement is a communication
problem it can be resolved by discussion between the nurse
(who must initiate the discussion) and the doctor (who must
be willing to explain the rationale and appreciate reasonable
suggestions). If the disagreement is between scientific
alternatives the "best" course can be defined by data, taking
into account the facilities available and the psychological
well-being of the patient. If the disagreement is based on
a value judgment, the person who disagrees must consider very
carefully whether his ethical or moral conviction is "better"
than that of the patient, or the doctor acting in behalf of
the patient.

If the patient disagrees with the doctor he can always

request more explanation or consultation (from a nurse or anyone else). If the disagreement persists, the patient can always choose another doctor or no doctor.

Troubling Problems in Medical Ethics: The Third
Volume in a Series on Ethics, Humanism, and Medicine: 203-205
© **1981 Alan R. Liss, Inc., 150 Fifth Ave., New York, NY 10011**

DISCUSSION SUMMARY: WHEN DOCTOR AND NURSE DISAGREE

Daria Chapelsky
CEHM
University of Michigan
Ann Arbor, Michigan

The majority of the participants generally agreed with
the speakers that the case depicted an ethical disagreement
between the doctor and nurse over personal value judgments
which ought to be resolved through appropriate communication.
However, like the speakers, the participants disagreed as to
whom the nurse should approach initially and the manner in
which she ought to communicate her concerns. The groups
were divided equally in support of each speaker.

All thirteen discussion groups concentrated on deriving
general principles from the concepts introduced by each
speaker, and from the specific questions posed in the case.
Using these principles as a framework, the participants then
formulated three alternatives available to the nurse (Elizabeth
Cornwall) in order to resolve this ethical conflict. The
nurse could either first approach the director of nursing
and chief resident (Dr. Manning) with her concerns, or
proceed with full disclosure to the patient's family, or
remain neutral and possibly withdraw from the case.

Five groups voted that the best alternative would be
for Miss Cornwall to approach the director of nursing and
Dr. Manning to obtain further information and clarification
of the case through open communication between doctor
and nurse. They based this decision on the premise that the
nurse's primary obligation is to follow the orders of her
supervisors. If the nurse remained dissatisfied with the
results of this approach, some participants suggested she
should then approach Mr. Schneider to encourage him to
obtain more information. Members of these groups agreed

that the family is entitled to various professional opinions
from different perspectives regarding the course of treatment. However, they insisted that Miss Cornwall's decision
to approach the family should not supersede or disobey the
director of nursing's orders. If the director of nursing
felt that approaching the family would disrupt the patient-
physician trust and collaborative team practice, then the
participants felt that Miss Cornwall should obey her and
abstain from approaching the family.

The second alternative suggested was for the nurse to
approach the patient's family directly, even without permission from her superviors. Most of the participants in five
other groups argued in support of this plan on the basis of
the nurse's personal and professional obligations. They
were particularly influenced by the ANA Code of Ethics,
which states that the nurse's primary obligation is to the
patient and not to the physician. This is held to supersede the nurse's contractual obligations to follow the
orders of physicians or supervisors. The participants
therefore felt that the nurse has the right to inform Mr.
Schneider about his wife's grave condition and to suggest
that he may request that the doctor discontinue treatment
and place Mrs. Schneider on "No Code" status. Several
participants stressed the importance of the nurses's personal
and profession obligations to use her own morality and
judgment in making such decisions in the best interest of
her patient. One participant suggested that the failure to
follow her own moral judgment might be viewed as an act of
ethical negligence.

The third option discussed was for the nurse to remain
neutral and to withdraw from the case if she felt sufficiently
uncomfortable with the physician's orders. Three groups
supported this as a reasonable alternative to intervention
by the nurse if communication with her supervisors had been
unsuccessful. Several participants in these groups disagreed, however, suggesting that if Miss Cornwall withdrew,
she might then be passively endorsing the physician's orders
and allowing the perceived medical wrong to continue.
Another participant suggested that the nurse might thereafter
choose to be employed in a situation that is more consistent
with her values so that she can either avoid these problems
in the future or resolve them more satisfactorily.

Several other ideas also evolved from the discussion

regarding how the nurse should act in attempting to resolve
the ethical dilemma. One popular suggestion was that the
nurse should initiate conferences among the health care team
and the patient's family. As "prophylactic ethics", some
participants suggested the development of a Hospital Ethics
Committee to evaluate patients' quality of life and to
resolve ethical dilemmas through discussion. Other discussants
suggested encouraging nurses to "learn ethics" and to "recognize the hospital's ethics code."

Troubling Problems in Medical Ethics: The Third
Volume in a Series on Ethics, Humanism, and Medicine: 207-208
© 1981 Alan R. Liss, Inc., 150 Fifth Ave., New York, NY 10011

INTRODUCTION: DOCTOR DRAFT: REDISTRIBUTING PHYSICIANS

Barbara Weil
Assistant Director for Publicity, CEHM
University of Michigan
Ann Arbor, Michigan

Judging from the present distribution of doctors, the
only people who need health care are those who live in urban
areas.   There are 198 practicing physicians per 100,000
people in New York State; South Dakota has 78.   Owyhee
County in Idaho, with a land area larger than the state of
Connecticut, has no practicing physicians, nor is it served
by a hospital.   In fact, 0.2% of our total population live
in counties lacking even one patient-care physician.

Why does this maldistribution exist, and what can be
done to remedy the situation? Lance Stell offers a partial
explanation: physicians' preferences about climate, recreational facilities, contact with other doctors, and
proximity to medical centers play a large part in their
choosing a place to practice.   Rural counties have very
little to offer in the way of medical facilities.

The case presented for discussion offers four possible
remedies, all of which utilize some form of compulsory
redistribution of physicians.   Bill A, while patterned after
Great Britain's Health Service, is partially based on the
Health Service Act, HR 2969, introduced by Hon Ronald V.
Dellums (D-CA).   This Act, one of many National Health
Insurance proposals before Congress, is unique because it
mandates a redistribution of future medical school graduates.
Under Dellum's proposal, a health care trainee would be
trained in his/her area at public expense, in return for a
term of service in a National Health Service facility.   The
service obligation would be equal to the length of the
student's medical education.

Dr. Joanne Lukomnik agrees with the Dellums plan, dismissing the notion of a 'draft'. Redistribution, she argues, is "a contractual agreement between people who choose certain types of education and what they would perform later." What is represented as a 'doctor draft' is actually salaried employment where a demand for physicians exists. Dr. Lukomnik's argument is based on the premise that other professionals go where the jobs are, and therefore, physicians should not be treated any differently than other American workers.

Lance Stell takes the opposing position, that an individual's actions are his property in a moral sense. Stell dismisses the 'right' of society to redistribute physicians. "Unless some account is given about how 'we' have acquired ownership rights of the actions of physicians, discussion of how 'we' ought to distribute their services is moot." Those who would order physicians to practice in certain areas fail to take doctors' rights seriously, and Stell contends that "People's lives are not social resources about which it is appropriate to ask, 'how ought they to be distributed?'" Since the Constitution prohibits involuntary servitude, except as punishment, Stell concludes that the protections of the Fourteenth Amendment prohibit the government from 'drafting' anybody, no matter what their profession.

REFERENCES

Blumberg MS (1971). "Trends and Projections of Physicians in the United States 1967-2002." Berkeley: The Carnegie Commission on Higher Education.
"Interim Report of the Graduate Medical Education National Advisory Committee to the Secretary, Dept. of Health, Education, and Welfare April 1979." Washington, D.C.: HEW, 1979. "National
"National Health Service Corps Scholarship Program: 1978-1979 Report to Congress." Washington, D.C.: HEW, 1978.

Troubling Problems in Medical Ethics: The Third
Volume in a Series on Ethics, Humanism, and Medicine: 209–211
© 1981 Alan R. Liss, Inc., 150 Fifth Ave., New York, NY 10011

DOCTOR DRAFT: REDISTRIBUTING PHYSICIANS

CASE FOR DISCUSSION

The Senate subcommittee on health care delivery is
concluding its long weeks of hearings on several proposed
bills for redistributing physicians to rural and under-
staffed urban areas. Several special-interest groups have
lobbied strongly in favor of at least one of the proposed
bills while the American Medical Association and many members
of the medical community have spoken out against the proposals. Three bills presently lie before the committee along
with a fourth which has been supported by a substantial
minority of physicians.

Bill A proposes a system of socialized medicine somewhat similar to that of Great Britain. All hospitals and
clinics would be offered the options of joining the American
Health Service (AHS) or surviving without government funding
or insurance payments. Medical schools and training schools
for other health professionals would have a similar choice,
with research grants and capitation (tuition assistance)
funds being awarded only to member schools. Schools, hospitals, and clinics wishing to remain outside the AHS could
do so if they could find private support funds or survive on
private patients' fees. The AHS would have the option of
establishing its own educational or health care facilities
as needed to provide appropriate health care and training.

Students attending AHS schools would pay no tuition and
would receive a small allowance for their living expenses
while in school. They would then be required to train in
AHS institutions and to work for the AHS after completion of
postgraduate training for two years or (for non-physicians)

for a length of time equivalent to their AHS education, not
to exceed two years. They would be paid salaries comparable
to non-medical civil servants of similar education and
training during this time and would have the option thereafter of remaining within the AHS and the civil service.
Alternatively, they could try to support themselves within
the private sector. Students attending non-AHS schools would
receive no federal scholarships, loans, or capitiation.
States would be urged to withdraw their subsidies. This
would require the average non-AHS medical student to pay
approximately $20,000 per year in tuition. NonAHS students,
like those already in practice at the time of enactment of
Bill A, would have the options of staying in the private
sector or signing up for the AHS at any time.

Bill B would continue the present level of government
capitation, financial aid, and student loan programs for
health care trainees, with an annual increase to keep pace
with costs. Additional funds would be made available for
financial aid grants. After residency training, all physicians
who had entered medical school after Bill B's enactment
would be sent to practice for two years wherever the National
Health Service Corps required them. Other trainees and
medical students already attending school would be required
to serve for an equivalent period of time (not to exceed two
years) to the time they had benefited from Bill B's financial
aid provisions. After fulfillment of the Bill B service
requirement, the physician or nurse could practice where he
or she wanted, although Bill B's sponsors hope that many
will stay where they had been placed. Refusal to meet the
service requirement of Bill B may be punished by fines of up
to $50,000 and up to one year in jail, although the National
Health Service Corps is granted the option of waiving all or
part of the requirement for special circumstances. Such
waivers are not to exceed ten students per year. Married
couples are to be placed together without requiring a
waiver.

Bill C is limited to physicians. It proposes that the
government pay for all medical education for all students
admitted to medical school, without dictating where these
students study. In return, all physicians would be required
to work in a salaried position for two years after residency,
placed by a National Health Board who would be notified of
health care shortages by regional boards. Following their
terms of service, doctors would be free to remain with the

Health Board or to go wherever they wish to practice. A medical student may be exempted from service by paying the government back for his education, with interest and allowing for inflation. (The government currently pays approximately 75% of all costs of education for a medical student. This would therefore come to about $60,000.)

Bill D would double the National Health Service Corps's current allocation with the stipulation that this additional money be used only to increase National Health Service Corps physician salaries and to pay for more National Health Service Corps scholarships to medical students (which require medical service after graduation).

Because of the unusual amount of controversy surrounding the debate, the subcommittee has gone into private session and parliamentary procedure has been suspended for the next hour. The Chairman bangs her gavel for silence and summarizes each bill. The subcommittee has been charged with either rejecting all the bills or endorsing no more than one as optimal. The Chairman has ruled that no further amendments will be accepted at this time, although you are welcome to offer them at the meeting of the main committee or on the Senate floor.

How do you vote? To what extent is your vote influenced by the right to health care? Do you believe such a right exists? How important is it in relation to the autonomy of health care professionals? If you feel unhappy with all of the proposals, is there an amendment you can offer at the next set of hearings which would substantially improve one of the bills? Is a two tier system of health care fair to the patients who cannot afford to enter the private sector? To health care professionals who cannot afford to buy their way out of the public sector? Is it fair to apply such a bill to health care professionals without including lawyers and teachers? To apply it only to doctors and ignore nurses and dentists? (What moral standards do you apply here in judging what is fair?)

(Case prepared by Barbara Weil and Marc D. Basson.)

Troubling Problems in Medical Ethics: The Third
Volume in a Series on Ethics, Humanism, and Medicine: 213-225
© **1981 Alan R. Liss, Inc., 150 Fifth Ave., New York, NY 10011**

STOP THE DRAFT: WHY COMPULSORY REDISTRIBUTION OF PHYSICIANS
WOULD BE WRONG

Lance K. Stell

Davidson College

Davidson, NC

THE QUESTION:

Should legislation be passed which requires physicians
to relocate their practices where government officals tell
them to? Should publicly funded medical schools be permitted
to educate only those students who are agreeable to having
officials restrict the range of choices about where they shall
practice? These questions must strike most of us as prepos-
terous for it seems possible to entertain them only if one
is prepared to abandon the cardinal values upon which our
political culture was founded - life, liberty and the pursuit of happiness.

To be sure, there are countries in which a citizen's
decisions about where he will work are subject to official
review and occasional veto, but it seems a low risk judgment
to claim that few people in our society identify with political systems where such practices are commonplace.

However, we must be careful not to hastily dismiss those
who believe that a positive answer to these questions merits
serious consideration. Rhetorically, it may be a good strategy
to disparage unliked ideas by associating those who advocate
them with bad company. Philosophically, such a strategy can
never be respectable for it is nothing more than a crude ad
hominem. People who believe in the rightness of compulsory
redistribution of physicians ought not be dismissed on the
grounds that such policies are practiced in countries where
general respect for rights we take for granted is lacking.
Presumably even the worst of places may have some wise

practices and reflective persons should appreciate them quite apart from other policies which are objectionable. More important still, a policy of compulsory redistribution may be justified if it is true, as some people think, that all citizens have a right to equal access to medical care (and that what prevents the exercise of it is a maldistribution of physicians rather than, say, a sheer shortage of them). One way to test whether a general right of a certain sort exists is to ask whether it would be unjust to do what the purported right implies or calls for. If so doing would be unjust, then the so-called right is no right at all. So the idea of mandatory redistribution of physicians provides a negative moral test for assessing the claim that a general right to equal access to medical care exists. It is not a full test because it is only a necessary condition of something's being a genuine right that it not be unjust to do what it implies. Therefore, we should examine the state of affairs which animates proposals for compulsory distribution of physicians and then move to an evaluation of the arguments which might be offered in support of such a policy. Along the way it will be important for me to sketch the theory of political morality to which I subscribe for only then will it be clear why the moral judgments I make come out as they do.

Without a moral theory to guide our reasoning and judgment, we have no grounds for assessing whether our beliefs about what ought or ought not to be done have any merit. Without a moral theory, we have no way of knowing whether what we are inclined to say about the situation is merely idiosyncratic to the way we have been socialized to think. For example, the intuitions of most people lead them to favor a rise in the general level of education in our country even though we can predict that an increase in the suicide rate will follow. On the other hand, these same people have intuitions that it would be wrong to experiment on and perhaps kill the feeble-minded in cancer research.[1] Can both judgments be coherently affirmed? Without a moral theory we cannot tell.

The political morality to which I subscribe can be broadly characterized as rights-based and liberal. Rights-based theories are a species of deontological theories of obligation all of which deny that the only morally relevant criterion for evaluating the rightness of a social policy is the comparative amount of good it may be expected to do.

The sacrifice of a minority to the interests of a majority is not made right by the greater net advantage. Each individual has rights which make it wrong to do certain things to him even though a collective gain would be thereby achieved. The position is liberal because of the way it distributes the burden of justification on proposals that would take away personal liberty, as well as for the way it describes how this burden must be born. It says that those who would restrict liberty bear the burden of showing that there exists a right that liberty be restricted in the way proposed. Additional features of the political morality to which I subscribe will emerge in the ensuing discussion.

For simplicity's sake, I will refer to proponents of mandatory distribution of physicians as "Drafters" and those who oppose the idea as "Dodgers." I think that the labels I have given the basic positions are equally unattractive so that no emotive advantage has been secured to either side in the distribution of names. For reasons to be explained below, the Drafters' strategy will be to show that considerations of social justice require a policy of compulsory distribution of physicians. The Dodgers' strategy whose part I shall be taking will be not only to block the Drafters' attempt but to show that the policy proposal is unjust.

THE PROBLEM

Enormous sums are spent on health care in the United States. In 1979 expenditures reached $212.2 billion or 9% of GNP.[2] According to government estimates, approximately $230 billion was spent on it last year - roughly 10% of GNP. Only in the category of defense do federal expenditures exceed those for health care. Costs are high for the average American as well. He spends the equivalent of one month's pay for medical insurance, physician's bills and hospital stays.

Despite these sizeable aggregate expenditures, the distribution of health care professionals and primary care facilities is very uneven. A study published by the AMA makes possible some striking illustrations of this point.[3] At the time of the study, two counties were singled out for dubious distinction. Owyhee County, Idaho, with its 7,641 square miles, was the largest United States county served by neither a physician nor a hospital. Osage County, Missouri,

with its 11,300 citizens, was the most populous United States
county not served by a patient care physician.[4] Although
Owyhee County is larger than Connecticut or Rhode Island or
Delaware, its population of 6,000 does not approach Connecticut's 3,000,000 plus. Connecticut by contrast had 5,341
patient care physicians and 10,763 hospital beds.[5] To match
Connecticut's physician-patient ratio of 573 : 1 our Idaho
county would have needed not one or two physicians but 10 or
11.

At the time of the study, Owyhee County's plight was
shared by 138 counties. Altogether they amounted to 148,426
squared miles (an area slightly larger than Montana) with a
population of 487,200. Thus 4.2% of the land area and 0.2%
of the total population are not served by a single patient
care physician.[6]

Even though one out of every seven new jobs created
between 1970 and 1977 was in the health care industry and the
past decade has seen a 25% increase in the number of active
physicians per 10,000 of population, there has been no
appreciable change in the uneven distribution of health care
professionals.[7] From 1970 to 1976 the number of physicians
in rural counties increased 16% and the physician-to-population ratio increased 6.7%. But during the same period, the
number of physicians in urban counties increased 24.8% and
the physician-to-population ratio increased 18.1%.[8] In 1978
the physician-to-patient ratio in non-metropolitan areas was
7.4 per 10,000 population, while the ratio was 17.1 per
10,000 population in metropolitan areas.[9]

A complete explanation for the uneven distribution would
be a formidable undertaking, but it seems obvious that at
least part of the explanation lies in the preferences
physicians weigh in selecting a location for their practices.
In a study conducted by the AMA and the Rand Corporation
physicians who graduated from medical school in 1965 were
surveyed concerning factors which influenced their location
choices. Seventy percent of the respondents mentioned climate
or geographical considerations, 63% cited the opportunity for
regular contact with other physicians, 62% cited the availability of clinical support facilities and personnel, 56%
cited availability or recreational and sports facilities and
55% cited the opportunity for regular contact with a medical
school or medical center.[10] The majority did not mention
per capita income as a factor but there is an obvious corre-

lation between the factors mentioned by the majority of the
respondents and per capita income. Per capita income is
some 80% higher in Connecticut than in Owyhee County.

The federal government and some state governments have
tried to make the distribution of physicians less uneven by
employing various incentive programs.[11] Some of these have
offered to forgive loans for capitation expenses to individuals
who were willing to serve where need was judged greatest.
Other programs have offered subsidies to medical schools
which would increase their enrollments, in the hope that the
disparity in distribution would be alleviated by increasing
the aggregate supply of physicians. Not only have these
schemes failed to make a noteworthy impact upon the uneven
distribution of physicians, the former sort has been criticized for having a discriminatory effect upon minorities who,
because of their comparatively low income backgrounds, are
disproportionally tempted by the lure of loan repayment
waivers.

SOME MORAL BACKGROUND

Some of those who are inclined to support the Drafters
on the question at hand may think that the data alone provide
sufficient grounds to justify a policy of compulsory distribution of physicians. To think this is a mistake. What if
anything should be done legislatively cannot be settled
until we are provided with an argument some of the premises
of which must be normative. These premises must say what
makes it right to pass laws of the sort proposed.

If assessing the moral/political issues between the
Drafters and the Dodgers we must be careful to note what is
not an issue between them. The issue which divides them is
not whether it is desirable for sick people to receive the
benefits health care professionals can provide. All sides
can agree that this is a good thing. The disagreement comes
over the question whether it is right to distribute the
people who provide the services in a more or less compulsory
way. From saying that something is a good thing or that
something should occur it does not follow that there is
justification to use the coercive instruments of law to bring
it about. Therefore, our moral deliberations about the
matter must be regulated by principles which differ from the
standards of decency and goodness which we commonly use to

evaluate the conduct and character of persons. Since we are
debating the merits of a social policy proposal, we must use
principles which are directed to the proper exercise of the
coercive powers of government.

Because the cardinal virtue of political institutions is
justice, the optimal strategy for the Drafter would involve
his showing that the policy he favors is required by justice.
Just political institutions recognize, respect and protect
the rights which persons have. On the other hand, the Dodger
can prevail by showing that people have rights which would
be violated were the Drafter's policy to be enacted.

As a value, justice differs from other important moral
values like beneficence or kindness because of its distinctive
connection with law and the warrant to use force. If a person
has a valid claim of justice against his fellows, he may
appropriately demand satisfaction as his due and use the
force of the law to secure what is owed him. By way of contrast, demands for beneficence are inappropriate - people do
not have a general right to beneficence or kindness.

It may be that neither the Drafter nor the Dodger has
justice on his side. If justice were indifferent to both
sides then some other value would have to adjudicate the
matter--social utility perhaps. I mention this possibility
for the sake of those who may be dissatisfied with the position of both the Drafter and the Dodger as I present them.

THE ARGUMENT FROM NEED

The most direct route for the Drafters to take in defend-
ing the propriety of their proposal attempts to show that
people have rights to health care, the recognition of which
entitles them to the advocated reduction in physicians'
liberty to choose where they shall practice. The basic idea
is that having a need for the services of health care professional provides the ground for a right to them. Bernard
Williams in his well-known essay "The Idea of Equality"
establishes the right as follows:

> . . .the proper ground of distributing medical
> care is ill health: this is a necessary truth.
> Now in very many societies, while ill health
> may work as a necessary condition of receiving

treatment, it does not work as a sufficient
condition, since treatment costs money, and
not all who are ill have the money; hence the
possession of sufficient money becomes in
fact an additional necessary condition of
actually receiving treatment. Yet more
extravagantly, money may work as a sufficient
condition by itself, without any medical
need, in which case the reasons that actually
operate for the receipt of this good are just
totally irrelevant to its nature; however,
since only a few hypochondriacs desire treatment when they do not need it, this is, in
this case a marginal phenomenon.

When we have a situation in which, for
instance, we can once more apply the notions
of equality and inequality: not now in
connection with the inequality between the
well and the ill, but in connection with the
inequality between the rich ill and the poor
ill, since we have straightforwardly the
situation of those whose needs are the same
not receiving the same treatment, though the
needs are the grounds of the treatment. This
is an irrational state of affairs.[12] (p. 163)

Although Williams limits himself to criticizing wealth
as a factor in receiving needed care, we should be confident
that he would find geographical consideration irrelevant as
well--especially given the high correlation between those
areas which are underserved and their comparatively low per
capita income. We can reformulate the argument as follows:

1. In distributing our benefits, persons have a
    right to be treated equally unless there is
    a relevant difference between them.

2. In distributing health care the only relevant
    criterion is the need for it.

3. Therefore, every American who needs the
    service of health care professionals is
    entitled to it irrespective of where he lives
    or what his income.

This argument plus the normative premise that it is right to use the force of the law to secure that to which people have rights together with additional factual premises drawn from the AMA study mentioned earlier would yield the conclusion that compulsory redistribution of physicians is justified.

The first premise requires clarification. We must distinguish between treating people identically and treating them as equals. The principle should not be understood as requiring that everyone be treated as if they were indistinguishable from each other. It requires that in distributing our benefits, we make the same relative contribution to the welfare of each person unless we have a relevant reason not to. We should notice too that the principle applies to the distribution of benefits which are truly ours to distribute. This may seem an obvious point but it often becomes lost when there is a slide from using the editorial "we" to the plural possessive "our." Presumably we ought not to accomplish by linguistic legerdermain something which needs a moral defense, viz., that the good we seek to "distribute" is really ours in the moral sense. When we speak about medical care the point becomes crucial because the object of discussion is a service activity--the actions of people. I should think that a person's actions morally belong to him and that some account must be given to establish that the ownership of them has passed (wholly or in part) to others. The presumption that a person's actions are his own makes it possible for us to understand how the voluntary acts he performs and the commitments he-makes bind him morally. It makes it possible for us to distinguish between a person's being obligated to do something and his being merely obliged to do it as when he is a captive or under extortionary threat. Unless some account is given about how "we" have acquired ownership rights of the actions of physicians, discussion of how "we" ought to distribute their services is moot.

The second premise is dubious for other reasons for it seems to appeal to an essentialist idea that certain human activities have a natural end or an internal goal and that the activity's legitimacy derives from the extent to which it produces (or tries to produce) the good it naturally aims at. Even if we grant that medical care has the restoration and/or preservation of health as its natural end, why should this take precedence over the purposes health care professionals may have in performing their work? Why should a physician's purposes of gaining wealth, recognition and self-fulfillment through the sale of his skills be less legitimate than the goal of making sick people well?[13] Why should the preferences physicians have which influence their choices about where to locate their practices be subordinated to the preferences of others who would have them do otherwise?

THE DRAFTER COUNTERATTACKS

For the moment, begins the Drafter, let it be granted that in the case of persons generally and physicians specifically the actions of the individual belong to him--that he is the owner of them in the moral sense. From the fact that a person's actions belong to him it does not follow that he is immune to moral constraints unless he consents to them. A person is not permitted to do whatever he wants with his property nor may he perform whatever acts he pleases. For example, he is not permitted to act in such a way that his acts bring harm to unconsenting second and third parties. This is not to say that people must have as the dominant goal of their activities the avoidance of harm; it means that the prohibition to harm serves as a kind of side constraint on their acts. Speaking very roughly and I suspect uncontroversially, it is a valid non-consensual principle that you may act in any way you choose provided that you not harm others who have not given their consent to risk harm at your hands.

In the case of professional licensure by society consensual principles do come into play. The control over certain kinds of activities is secured to professionals as a monopoly but in exchange for this public grant comes the correlative duty not to engage in the activity in ways that are contrary to the public good. Might it not be the case that in making decisions about where to locate their practices in the way they do, physicians are illegitimately ignoring their part of the bargain? In the survey about factors which influence a physician's decision about where to locate his practice, there was no mention by a majority of those surveyed that the public good was a factor which influenced their decision about where they would locate their practices. Since physicians have shown themselves on balance to be morally blind to their duty not to act contrary to the public good it falls now to the law to remind them of this.

Furthermore, says the Drafter, your categorical assumption that a person's acts belong to him is highly dubious at least in connection with those performed in his capacity as a health care professional. Medical knowledge emerges as a product of social cooperation. Since medical knowledge is produced socially it is appropriate that society retain control over who will have this knowledge, where and how it will be applied. Thus a different metaphor seems called for. Rather than the owner of his acts, we should see the physician as a trustee of a public good (medical knowledge) which makes his activities as a physician possible. Ownership of the knowledge rests with society which retains a veto over decisions which the physicians may make--specifically those about where he locates his practice.[14]

THE DODGER DODGES

Four different responses must be made to the Drafter's view. First we must call to mind a distinction which his position ignores--the distinction between harming and failing to benefit. When an M.D. upon completing his residency in Ann Arbor decides to enter practice in Marin County, California, his decision does no harm to the citizens in Osage County, Missouri, or Owyhee County, Idaho. His decision causes them no loss; they have no complaint against him. His decision fails to benefit them but they have no right to benefit from him. Absent the existence of special obligations, there simply is no right to beneficence.

The second point concerns the monopoly physicians enjoy because of the certification and licensing procedure. If it is true that accepting this benefit carries with it obligations to serve the common good, how or better who should determine when this duty is being discharged properly? The common good is a blank check with near limitless draw on the public power to underwrite all sorts of tyrannical interventions with individual liberty. More to the point is the question whether there is justification for the state to create such monopolies in the first place. Monopolies always function to restrict supply and raise price--but this is a matter which would occasion a lengthy discussion.

The third comment concerns the idea that medical knowledge is socially produced and so socially owned. Take first the idea that knowledge is produced socially. If it

makes any sense at all to speak about knowledge as a product
resulting from social cooperation, it is a product in a very
different sense than automobiles or televisions are social
products. Marxists may strike a respondant chord when they
speak about the process of expropriating the product from
those who produced it but what sense does it make to say this
about knowledge? If I learn and hence come to know what you
know, you have not lost any of what you had. What you have may
now be worth less (i.e., not command as high a price) than
before because there are now more people to service any
available demand. Knowledge is not intrinsically scarce.
Indefinitely many people may acquire it and apply it for their
own purposes without using it up. Besides, our social legacy
is composed not only of much knowledge but much foolishness
as well. Unfortunately, those who perpetuate the legacy do
not conform to the highest standards of "truth in labeling."
In any event, a person is no more justified in attempting to
extract compensation from society for whatever ill the foolishness may have done him than society is justified in holding him up for any benefits he may have derived from the
knowledge. The knowledge that a person possesses is a subset
of his beliefs (the true ones). How can it be that beliefs
which I have belong to someone else in the moral sense? It
is true that we think of plagiarism as the theft of someone
else's ideas but we may avoid wrongdoing even here by
acknowledging that the ideas were originally produced by
someone else. In fact we would think it odd if the origina-
tor of an idea insisted that we give his idea back to him
and we should be positively amused were he to insist that
we forget his idea. For these reasons, it seems bizarre
to think of knowledge as property at all--social or individual.

Finally and most seriously, the position of the Drafter
must be rejected because it fails to take seriously the
underlying fact which gives a rights-based theory its point,
viz., that each of us is an individual with his own life to
live. Our lives do not constitute mere possible sensations
in some corporate consciousness, nor are they candidates for
possible inclusion in a broader collective experience. To
take rights seriously is to be offended at the suggestion
that people's lives are social resources which can be
"distributed" evenly or unevenly. Rights protect the
separateness of our several existences, morally shielding
us from invasions and appropriations by collections of
other individuals who would surely win if outcomes were
appropriately settled by counting sums. Justice refuses to

allow that the sacrifices imposed on a few may be legitimately offset by marginal gains enjoyed by others.

WILLING COMPLIANCE WITH THE UNENFORCEABLE

I want to conclude by doing two things: refocus the precise nature of the problem under discussion; attack a sort of moral smugness which may draw unintended and unjustified reinforcement for insensitivity to human need. First I reiterate that the issue under discussion is a political question and as such must be answered by the principles of a political morality. A political morality seeks to regulate the interaction between the citizen and his government by formulating principles which separate those uses of public power which are justified from those which are not. The political morality to which I have appealed is rights-based. It says that the citizen has rights which trump social policy proposals to roll over his liberty even when there is a powerful case that the good of many others would be thereby served. Out Constitution embodies some of these by forbidding the government to use certain means in the pursuit of ends otherwise judged to be desirable. It imposes disabilities on government to repress freedom of speech and the publication of ideas. It forbids government to deny any citizen the equal protection of the laws and yes, it forbids involuntary servitude except as a punishment for crime. Now my own feeling is that the Thirteenth Amendment prohibits the government from "drafting" anyone. Making good on this claim would require an essay in its own right.

Finally, I address a few remarks to both the Drafter and the Dodger. To the Drafter, who probably thinks me mistaken, I ask that he produce the principle of his political morality which makes it right for government to use its coercive powers in the ways proposed. How, precisely, are those principles stated? What evidence is there that the good sought can be gotten in no other way? It is not enough to show that the good sought has not been achieved in other ways but that it could not be.

To those who, for reason of self-interest, tend to identify with the position of the Dodger, I wish to remind them that political morality is not the whole of morality. Political morality is essentially a crude instrument and so must ignore those sensitive areas of everyday life which are

concerned with the personal virtue of benevolence. A person
cannot infer that because he is not violating anyone's rights
that his conduct is morally unobjectionable--he may only infer
that his conduct is not unjust. We have moral duties to meet
the needs of others and to promote their good when so doing
does not result in zero-sum self-sacrifice. Principles of
personal morality require that we do the most marginal good.
The fact that our duties of beneficence are not enforceable
does not lessen their urgency. One should not infer that
the unenforceability of beneficence relegates it to the realm
of the superogatory. Those who are never benevolent do not
merely fail to be praiseworthy. Selfishness is a vice and
is properly condemned as a defect of the moral personality.
Thus a willingness to serve where needed does not elevate a
person into the rarefied atmosphere of the saints but rather
reflects a simple determination to love one's neighbor as
oneself.

1. This example from Philippa Foot (1980). "Virtues & Vices."
       Berkeley: University of California Press, p. 101.
2. "Health--United States 1980"(1980).Hyattsville, Maryland:
       U.S. Department of Health and Human Services, p. 101.
3. G. A. Roback (1974). "Distribution of Physicians in the
       U.S., 1973. Chicago: American Medical Association.
4. Ibid., p. 24.
5. Ibid., p. 20.
6. Ibid., p. 24.
7. "Health," Supra, p. 12.
8. Ibid., p. 79.
9. Ibid., p. 12.
10. Barry, S. Eisenberg, Ed. (1974). "Socioeconomic Issues
       of Health." Chicago: American Medical Association,
       pp. 40-1.
11. Ibid., pp. 42-48.
12. Bernard Williams (1969). "The Idea of Equality" in
       Joel Feinberg, ed., "Moral Concepts." New York:
       Oxford University Press, p. 163.
13. Robert Nozick (1974). "Anarchy, State and Utopia.
       New York: Basic Books, p. 234.
14. This is a version of an argument first put forward by
       Marx Wartofsky of Boston University. He develops the
       argument thoroughly and eloquently. See his paper
       in this volume.

Troubling Problems in Medical Ethics: The Third
Volume in a Series on Ethics, Humanism, and Medicine: 227–234
© **1981 Alan R. Liss, Inc., 150 Fifth Ave., New York, NY 10011**

REDISTRIBUTING PHYSICIAN SERVICES: SOME ETHICAL ISSUES

Joanne E. Lukomnik, M.D.

Associate Professor of Community Medicine,
Sophie Davis School of Biomedical Education,
City College of the City University of New York

...the truth is that medicine, professedly founded
on observation, is as sensitive to outside influences, political, religious, philosophical, imagi-
native, as is the barometer to the change of at-
mospheric density. Theoretically, it ought to go
on its own straightforward inductive path without
regard to changes of government or to fluctuations
of public opinion. But look a moment, while I
clash a few facts together, and see if some sparks
do not reveal by their light a closer relation
between the Medical Sciences and the conditions
of Society and the general thought of the time,
than would first be suspected.

> --Oliver Wendell Holmes
> Annual Discourse 1860
> Massachusetts Medical Society

The American Medical Association adopted its first
Principles of Medical Ethics in 1847; it began debate on the
latest revision in 1978. This code has provided physicians
with a guide to acceptable relationships among professionals
and with rules of membership into their professional guild,
but it has had little to say about the ethics of relationships with patients (Carleton B. Chapman, "On the Definition and Teaching of the Medical Ethic", New England Journal
of Medicine, Vol. 39, No. 12, Sept. 20, 1979). Such rules
of physician conduct, while necessary and useful for organizational and professional purposes, do not define the full
range of ethical and moral issues raised when professional

practice takes place. Approaches to that area of medical ethics, as opposed to the rules of a guild, may center around physician-patient rights and obligations, around an implied social contract between physicians as a whole and society, or as "guides to correct conduct derived from moral precepts but generally more restrictive and usually applied to [physicians] whose obligations to society are, because of the nature of their activities, different from those of the community as a whole" (Ballantine, 1979).

In what sense, then, is the subject of this discussion, the "doctor draft", an issue of medical ethics, and how shall we approach the discussion? Axiomatically, the manner in which we pose the question defines the domain of the answer. By defining the issue as "doctor draft", there is an implied assertion that there is a unique ethical dimension to the problem of physicians' services which is not inherent to the services provided by other health workers such as nurses, physical and occupational therapists, nutrition aides, and others who provide health care. Secondarily, by using the word "draft", a word which, in this country, and especially for those of us who reached draftable age during the Viet Nam War, is emotionally labeled, we immediately raise issues of an individual's obligation to his/her society and an individual's right and duty to resist a social obligation which the individual finds morally and ethically repugnant. The papers preceding this one indeed framed the issue as one involving draft and draft dodgers, but this is not the issue before us.

The problem, in its most simplified form, can be stated as: Given the maldistribution of physicians in this country, can and should government attempt to correct this maldistribution? Are proposals to correct such a maldistribution utilizing such methods as placing physicians in salaried employment or requiring physicians to serve an obligated period, either in an underserved geographic area or in an underserved specialty, in conflict with individual rights to choose to practice a profession solely in accord with individual preference?

Most health professionals are, in fact, in some kind of salaried employment. Most nurses, for instance, find employment wherever jobs are available after they finish nursing school. If necessary, they move to where there is

a job. Some nurses, it is true, choose not to take a salaried position and, in one form or another, depending on the
Nurse Practice Act in the state they are in, set up a private practice. If they do, for the most part they do not
have access to a hospital. Furthermore, if trained as an
intensive care unit nurse, there is little likelihood she
would be allowed to go into private practice in an ICU.

By posing the issue of possible solutions to the problem of physician maldistribution as one of "doctor draft",
one would implicitly support the claim for privileges that
doctors want for themselves, and that very few groups, other
than physicians, enjoy in this country. It is important to
try and understand why it is that we find posed as an "ethical" issue the question of whether doctors should be treated
like other health professionals. Is there something unique
about doctors, about the skills and the knowledge they have,
that implies they should have rights that no other health
professional claims, to locate where they wish, and to serve
those they choose to serve?

There are a number of reasons why medicine should be
a public function, with public responsibilities. First, the
medical profession is necessarily a monopoly in which the
practitioners, by virtue of their training, have access to
skills and information to which the public, the laity, has
no access except through the mediation and intervention of
the practitioners. Putting aside for the moment arguments
as to the efficacy of medical care, it can be argued that
to deny access to medical care is to deny a fundamental pre-
requisite to the optimal exercise of the right to life, liberty, and the pursuit of happiness.

Although one can claim there is public access to the
information that medical students receive--as is argued in
the preceding paper--realistically, access to medical education is limited and very expensive, even though much of
the cost is absorbed by the public realm. Well-documented
class and racial biases in admissions to medical schools
make it clear that "equal opportunity" has no applicability
here. It is naive and self-serving to argue that all patients
and consumers potentially have access to the same medical
knowledge and skills as physicians, merely by undertaking
an autodidactic course at their local library. Since physicians enjoy the practical monopoly of medical knowledge and
skills on the basis of their special training, we need to

look at the source of that training.

Medical education is, in fact, paid for mainly by public funds. In the past, a large amount of Federal money has gone into capitation funds to medical schools. Even though this form of financing is decreasing, other funds are replacing them--Federal research and education grants, faculty training grants, and state funds. The public's insurance monies go into maintaining the hospitals in which medical students train, and into paying for the care received by the patients in wards where they find training "material". Finally, many medical students today receive public scholarships. However, even when the individual pays tuition, this covers only a small portion of the total cost. All these other, public funds account for a large fraction of the total cost of medical education. In fact, in the country as a whole, about 78% of the support for medical schools is paid out of public funds.

Furthermore, physicians, when they finish their training, whether they serve in some public capacity or go into private practice, have regular access to hospitals where they can place their patients, treat them, and receive fees for this treatment--even though these institutions are generally built with public funds and receive much of their continuing financial support from public sources. Today approximately 50% of the operating funds of hospitals in this country--and this includes private and "voluntary" hospitals as well as public facilities--comes out of public funding.

One can point to analogous situations in other fields where such a privilege is absent. Teachers, for the most part, receive their education at publicly-supported institutions. Even when they pay tuition, a large part of their education is financed out of public funds. They have some choices when they finish, including teaching within public schools, teaching within private schools, or setting themselves up as tutors. If they do act as tutors--that is, go into "private practice"--they do not have access either to public or private schools, unless they arrange a specific contract with those institutions. Similarly, someone trained as a police officer can choose to serve within a jurisdiction which has a need for police officers or private security guards. If they choose to set up as private investigators, they do not have access to the resources, the facilities, or the equipment of the police department of that community. No one talks about a policeman as having been "drafted" into the police force or teachers as having been "drafted" into the school system; they have simply accepted a job where the jobs are.

Likewise, if I am an automobile worker in Flint, Michigan, and I would like to become a manager, no one holds that GM has to give me that job. In nearly every other field, there is a distribution of job opportunities which is controlled, in many different ways. The people who pay, generally corporate employers, decide what types of jobs should be available and what types of specialized training are needed to fit those jobs. In the case of medicine, the public, through its taxes, not only pays for the training of physicians, but also for their further specialty education and for the facilities they work in, but concedes to individual doctors the determination of where they should practice.

Do we discriminate against the physician if we decide that he or she must locate in an area where a job is available, and that the job's availability should depend on the need for physicians in that area? Again, that depends on how we pose the question. If we say we should "draft" physicians to force them to move to an underserved area, physicians would appear to be singled out for a burden not shared by the rest of society. If we say, on the other hand, that a job will be available in the same way that a job is available to a nurse, a teacher, a policeman, or an automobile factory worker, we will be looking at the problem in a totally different way.

Government intervention in distributing health resources, including physicians, would not be necessary if "competition" worked in the medical marketplace. Medical costs are rising, faster, even, than other prices. Because doctors have a monopoly, they can set their own fee scales. Indeed, many other costs within medicine can be shown to be tied to the ways in which doctors' fees are set so that, in fact, no free market operates within medicine today. Thus, anyone fortunate enough to be able to attend medical school is practically assured of financial success after graduation, a far different situation from that facing students in nearly any other field.

The rights of patients, as well as those of doctors, need to be included in this discussion. In examining the doctor's right to choose the area that he or she wants to practice in, the specialty he or she wants to practice, and the population he or she feels most comfortable with (generally, an upper-middle class population which can afford to bring the doctor's income up to what the doctor would like it to be), we cannot ignore the issue of the patient's right to choose. How free is the choice on the part of the average patient when the receipt of medical care depends on the ability to pay, the geographical area lived in, or the color of one's skin?

There is, in fact, a very much bigger medical maldistribution problem than has previously been suggested. Right now there are 1,800 Federally-designated Health Manpower Shortage Areas containing a population of 51 million people. Obviously, some of these people have access to medical care, but most have limited or no access to care. At this moment, by reports of the Graduate Medical Education National Advisory Committee (GMENAC), by AMA estimation for 1978, and by Department of Health and Human Services estimation, there is a need for at least 14,000 primary care physicians to provide an acceptable level of services in those areas.

The "free market" system has not solved that problem. Although there is some indication that pieces of the problem (e.g., the presence of specialists outside of metropolitan centers) are getting better, the overall picture is not getting very much better. Of the ten states that had the lowest physician/population ratio in 1950, seven were still among the lowest ten in 1977. Of the ten states that had the highest physician/population ratio in 1950, eight are still among the top ten. Fully 57% of poor rural counties had a physician/population ratio of less than 1:2000, while 45% of non-poor rural counties also had this extremely low physician/population ratio.

Furthermore, there is a maldistribution by specialty training as well as by geographic area. In 1971 approximately 6% of all rural counties did not have a primary care physician; in 1977, 6.3% of these counties did not have a primary care physician. Specialty training--which tends to take physicians out of primary care and into more population locations--is supported mostly out of public funds.

In defining the problem, not as one of "doctor draft",
but as whether there should be a public role, and a government role, in distributing physicians and medical care, both
by specialty and geographic location, to meet the needs of
this country at this time, I am raising a moral, social and
political question. Paraphrasing the utilitarian philosophical model, we can ask what route we should follow to achieve
the greatest good for the greatest number. If we merely continue to rely on the presumed virtue and good intentions of
individual physicians, the problems of access will be per-
petuated through another generation. Can we find a political
solution that meets public needs and does not violate individual rights?

Doctors should be trained at public expense, in return
for which the doctor would agree to practice where a job was
available and where his/her skills were needed. The community would support the physician, for some period of time,
at a reasonable salary. This is not a doctor draft. Indeed,
it is one method of redistribution which depends on a contractual understanding between the potential physician and
the society which supports his/her education.

Furthermore, a doctor who chooses, later, to go into
private practice and not to work for a salary would not be
able to use facilities that were supported by public funds.
If this were done, you would have done no differently than
when you say that someone who has trained as a teacher and
sets up as a private tutor may not use the classroom in the
public school.

This is not involuntary servitude, to say to someone
that, if you choose to go to medical school under public
auspices and with public funds, then you will practice, at
least for a period of time, in the public good. It is not
involuntary servitude to say that, if you have trained in
this fashion, you may still go into private practice, but
you may not have access to public facilities. I do not see
this as an abridgement of human or constitutional rights.

When we talk about life, liberty, and the pursuit of
happiness, which are, for all of us, things that we hold
dear, it is nowhere stated that any of us should become
wealthy at the public's expense--even if personal wealth
were our definition of happiness. Medicine is, in fact, a
public industry. It is 10% of our GNP, with about 8.5% of

that coming from the general public, either through government expenditures, tax credits, or insurance payments. No
one has guaranteed me that if I decide to set up a factory,
or work in one, or set up a school, or work in one, I can
use public money for my private pursuit of happiness.
Physicians should be treated no differently from any other
group of workers in this country.

REFERENCES

Ballantine HT Jr. (1979). The crisis in ethics anno
    domine 1979. NEJM 30(12).
Chapman CB (1979). On the definition and teaching of the
    medical ethic. NEJM 39(12).

Troubling Problems in Medical Ethics: The Third
Volume in a Series on Ethics, Humanism, and Medicine: 235–237
© **1981 Alan R. Liss, Inc., 150 Fifth Ave., New York, NY 10011**

DISCUSSION SUMMARY: DOCTOR DRAFT: REDISTRIBUTING PHYSICIANS

Barbara Weil
Assistant Director for Publicity, CEHM
University of Michigan
Ann Arbor, Michigan

None of the groups approved of any one bill unanimously, although the bill chosen most often in final votes was Bill D, which would offer physicians more attractive salaries as incentive to join the National Health Service Corps. Most groups began their discussion with the assumption that everyone has a right to health care, or at least that it would be a morally desirable thing for the government to ensure that a certain level of health care would be available for all. They therefore concluded that there is a need to move doctors and other health care professionals to underserved areas.

Other proposed bills were rejected for several reasons, the major one being that it was not fair to require only doctors (or only health care professionals as opposed to other professionals) to serve for two years in underserved areas. Some participants argued that a mandatory service requirement was an unfair restriction of choice, while others claimed that most underserved areas could not afford to support a private practice. Some participants objected to the likely loss of continuity in the doctor-patient relationship when the doctor left his assigned area after his service period. Others pointed out that most of the doctors in the underserved areas would be fresh out of residency when they served, with very few experienced doctors available for consultation. They wondered if such systems would lead to the provision of poor quality health care by inadequately experienced physicians in mandatory service regions.

Specifically, Bill A was rejected because it proposed a two-tier system of health care creating, as one participant commented, "a separate health care system for the super-rich." Another commented that it was absurd to cut off the private sector from public grants and thereby almost eliminate private research. The few participants who approved of this bill did so because it was voluntary and would drastically redistribute the provision of health care.

Bill B, requiring service from all health care trainees was disapproved of by all but two dissenters, who argued that it applied to all health care professionals and was therefore equitable. Objections to this bill included its mandatory nature, the placement of "green" doctors in under-served areas, and the requirement for service no matter who had paid for medical school.

Conversely, most participants rejected Bill C because wealthier students could "buy out" of the plan. Bill C also limited the service requirement to physicians which participants felt was not fair. C did receive more votes than A or B, because it did not dictate where a student must go to school, but rather offered free tuition as an incentive to work in underserved areas.

Bill D received the most votes; it was cited as "fairest" of the bills. Participants argued that if monetary incentives increased, so would the number of doctors in problem areas. Some persons objected to this bill on the grounds that the National Public Health Service Corps has been inadequate and inefficient and that increasing capitation would be "throwing good money after bad."

Several participants offered alternative suggestions for redistributing health care appropriately. These included the following:

Set up group practices in rural areas. This would provide the new doctor with peers for consultation, and would keep him from being overworked.

Accept or recruit more medical students from rural areas, and hope that they will return to practice there.

Wait for the expected glut of doctors in the 1990's, and

hope that the problem solves itself.

The participants ultimately agreed that, although patients have a right to health care, doctors have a more significant right to choose when and where to practice. This was their final reason for rejecting bills requiring medical service in favor of bills such as Bill D which only offer greater inducements to doctors who practice in underserved areas.

**Troubling Problems in Medical Ethics: The Third
Volume in a Series on Ethics, Humanism, and Medicine: 239–240
© 1981 Alan R. Liss, Inc., 150 Fifth Ave., New York, NY 10011**

INTRODUCTION: THE RIGHT TO PRIVACY WHEN LIVES ARE AT STAKE

Marc D. Basson
Director, CEHM
University of Michigan
Ann Arbor, Michigan

There is an old medical saying that all of medicine can
be learned from a single patient. A case such as this one
makes one wonder whether this proverb ought to be extended
to medical ethics as well. The case presented here was
originally conceived as pitting a deontological rights-
principle (that every person has the right to control information about him) against a horrible consequence, a death
that might be avoided if confidentiality were breached and
the tissue type of a possible bone marrow donor revealed.
We were attempting to make the point that deontological
principles are often only prima facie valid, that they can
properly be overridden by other ethically relevant aspects
of a situation. We were so certain that participants would
endorse the breach of privacy needed to save a girl's life
that we felt impelled to include elements of deceit and
coercion simply to provoke some controversy.

As will become shortly apparent to the reader, we
vastly underestimated the complexity of the case, for no
ethical question is simple. Arthur Caplan advances in his
discussion here powerful consequentialist arguments in
defense of honoring privacy. He suggests that if violations
of privacy are allowed to occur, they may become widespread
and that when non-physicians learn of them, such consequences
as the depletion of the human subject pool for experimentation
and serious harm to the doctor-patient relationship may
occur. These evils, he suggests, may far outweigh the loss
of one girl's life, particularly when we are not certain
that she can be saved. Caplan also reminds us that the
first step to resolving an ethical dilemma is often to

refuse to accept the terms in which it is described. Rather than accepting the case's implication that only Plantar can donate his bone marrow and save the patient's life, Caplan suggests alternative possibilities which ought to be explored.

Gerald Abrams adds still more complications in his paper. He reminds us of other violations of privacy that occur routinely in the medical setting, such as those necessary for medical education, suggesting that no moral principle can be as simple as "respect privacy always." Abrams also describes the consequentialist tradeoff between protection of privacy and ease of access to needed medical information that is defined by our current state of the art in in information processing. Protection, he reminds us, will cost time and money, and while psychiatric records may require elaborate safeguards, it may not be cost-effective to protect serum potassium levels and tissue types, even though the patient may be equally entitled to have these protected if he chooses. The general thrust of Abrams's paper is to challenge us to refine our principles and delineate our exceptions, to consider who, when, where, how, and why in addition to what before passing moral judgments. Yet, at the same time. Abrams points out the urgency of decision, for bone marrow donation seems likely to be a commonplace soon, and many decisions ought to be made beforehand.

The combinations of moral principles with consequences, individual cases with public policy implications, and above all complexity with urgency, all pervade this case and perhaps make it an especially appropriate topic with which to close this volume. Grappling with issues such as these is not only interesting and challenging, but necessary if medicine is to be practiced as it should be.

Troubling Problems in Medical Ethics: The Third
Volume in a Series on Ethics, Humanism, and Medicine: 241–243
© 1981 Alan R. Liss, Inc., 150 Fifth Ave., New York, NY 10011

THE RIGHT TO PRIVACY WHEN LIVES ARE AT STAKE

CASE FOR DISCUSSION

The intensity of chemoradiotherapy that is routinely
used in combatting leukemia is usually limited by bone
marrow toxicity. Bone marrow transplantation therefore
would permit more aggressive therapy, with transplanted
marrow replacing that destroyed by chemotherapy. Transplantation may also aid in killing any leukemic cells still
present. Bone marrow transplants between identical twins or
HLA-identical siblings for leukemia or aplastic anemia have
been fairly successful. Bone marrow transplants between
unrelated persons are currently not performed because of the
immunologic rejection of the transplant by the recipient.
However, just as kidney transplants have become possible
between two unrelated people, so someday non-related bone
marrow transplantation may also become possible. This case
is set in a year in the future in which bone marrow transplants between people who are not relatives can be successfully performed. It is therefore hypothetical, but the
ethical issues involved are nevertheless real and timely.
Please accept the hypothesis and concentrate on these
issues for the purposes of discussion.

Evon Fields is a bright ten year old girl with untreated,
newly diagnosed acute myelocytic leukemia (AML). The treatment of choice for Evon is total body irradiation and chemotherapy followed by a bone marrow transplantation from a
compatible donor. Of all her relatives, only Evon's Aunt
Karen would be a compatible donor. However, Karen refuses
to be the donor because although perfectly healthy, she
believes the risk to her would be too great.

Dr. Robb, Evon's doctor, knows of no one both eligible
and willing to be a donor. The doctor dispiritedly tells
her friend Dr. Krieger her problem. Krieger excitedly
recalls a research project he did last year which involved
HLA-typing of several hundred people. He locates his old
records and finds one suitable donor, Brian Plantar.

An appointment is set up between Mr. Plantar and Dr.
Robb after permission is obtained from the Fields family to
discuss Evon's case with potential donors. The doctor
explains to Mr. Plantar the circumstances of Evon's situation.
In addition, she says that the procedure of taking bone
marrow from a donor is performed under general anesthesia in
a sterile operating room. The technique is not difficult.
The bone marrow is obtained by approximately one hundred
punctures of the sternum (breastbone) and of the anterior
and posterior iliac crests (bones of the pelvis). Multiple
punctures are needed to maximize the number of bone marrow
cells obtained. From the punctures, between 500 and 750 ml
of blood and bone marrow are removed, processed, and then
immediately administered to the recipient in the ward.

In addition, Mr. Plantar is informed of the minimal
risks of the operation to the donor. There is 1/10,000
chance of death associated with the use of general anesthesia.
Less serious but slightly more likely risks include having a
heart attack from the stress of anesthesia, developing
aspiration pneumonitis, incurring damage to the teeth from
intubation, and developing such minor postoperative reactions
as headaches, nausea, vomiting, dizziness, and weakness.
Also associated with surgery is a small chance of the patient
developing an infection or a bleeding problem. During the
removal of the bone marrow, a unit of blood that was taken
from the donor a few days previously is given back to the
donor. This "autotransfusion" eliminates many of the normal
risks of blood transfusion for the donor. Mr. Plantar is
also told that some of the puncture sites may be sore for a
few days after the operation. The loss of some bone marrow
does not present any problems for the donor because he has a
sufficient reserve and because bone marrow regenerates
itself.

Dr. Robb also comments on the potential risks and
benefits of the bone marrow transplant for the recipient.
The recipient of a bone marrow transplant is exposed to the
risk of developing graft-versus-host disease, which can be a

fatal complication. He also increases his chances of developing severe infections, especially pneumonia. However, the
potential benefits of a transplantation for the recipient
far surpass the risks. Chemotherapy combined with bone
marrow transplantation offers the possibility of longterm
remission or cure in the majority (over 60%) of the patients
who receive transplants during the first remission of the
AML. (Thomas, et al., 1979). It is unlikely that a significant rate of longterm remission or cure could be achieved
in AML without bone marrow transplantation.

Dr. Robb then asks Mr. Plantar if he has any questions.
The doctor tells Mr. Plantar that he is under no obligation
to make the donation, but reminds him that he is the only
tissue-matched donor available to Evon. (No mention is made
of Evon's Aunt Karen.) Dr. Robb concludes by showing him
Evon's picture and asking him to think matters over.

Was it improper of Dr. Krieger to offer his research
files to help find a bone marrow donor? Given that Dr.
Krieger made the offer to disclose information from his
research, was it unethical of Dr. Robb to accept it? Does
Mr. Plantar have the opportunity for informed and uncoerced
consent? Does Mr. Plantar have a right to privacy which
extends to his HLA-haplotype? Has it been violated in this
case? If so, does the need to treat Evon in the manner
proposed take precedence over Mr. Plantar's right to privacy?
How does the existence of a potential related donor who has
refused affect the case? Would your decision be different
if Mr. Plantar was himself a patient of Dr. Robb?

(Case prepared by Laurie Winkelman and Marc D. Basson.)

Troubling Problems in Medical Ethics: The Third
Volume in a Series on Ethics, Humanism, and Medicine: 245–255
© **1981 Alan R. Liss, Inc., 150 Fifth Ave., New York, NY 10011**

THE RIGHT TO PRIVACY WHEN LIVES ARE AT STAKE

Arthur L. Caplan
Associate for the Humanities
The Hastings Center
360 Broadway
Hastings-on-Hudson, New York

Oftentimes people faced with the prospect of reading a philosophical paper in medical ethics complain that such papers never provide any answers. However, the value of having simple answers to hard moral questions is, I believe, highly overestimated. Consider these 'expert' moral answers to the questions raised in our case study:

Was it or is it improper for the researcher to offer access to research records in order to locate this donor?
Answer, almost certainly it was wrong.

Was it unethical of the little girl's doctor to accept the offer of the information once the search had been made?
Answer, almost certainly it was wrong.

Does the identified donor have the opportunity for a free consent to the donation?
Answer, no, not under the conditions described in this case.

Do persons have a right to privacy over their HLA haplotypes?
Answer, yes.

Has privacy been violated in this case?
Answer, yes.

Whose rights take precedence in this case, donor or
recipient?
Answer, as the case is given, the donor's.

How does the existence of another donor affect the
case?
Answer, the existence of the other donor in the case
makes a big moral difference; it makes the behavior in
the case unethical.

There are some simple and plain moral answers. It
should be obvious that these answers require reasons to be
convincing. It is the reasons, principles, and the analysis
motivating any moral point of view that makes moral answers
interesting. Since this is so, I will organize my presentation around three main themes. First, the identification
of some ethical issues raised by certain role conflicts in
the case. I shall discuss three professional roles where
moral issues arise: the researcher/patient relationship,
the doctor/patient relationship, and the society/doctor
relationship. Next, having examined those relationships
and what they mean for assessing the behavior that went on
in this case, I will inquire into some general ethical
issues concerning voluntary organ donation. Finally, I shall
present a set of necessary conditions for conducting donations in the area of organ and tissue gifts in an ethical
manner.

I.   TRANSPLANTATION AND THE DUTIES OF PHYSICIANS

A. The Ethics of the Researcher/Subject Relationship

In the case, the researcher, Dr. Krieger, who is a
friend of Dr. Robb, the physician in charge of the little
girl's care, makes information available about an identifiable person to another physician. As noted above, I think
this act is morally wrong. Why?

The researcher/subject relationship is a contractual
relationship. It is based on promises. Under the present
regulations governing the activity of human experimentation,
people must participate voluntarily in research (Capron,
1974). Their voluntary participation is obtained by guaran-
teeing that their privacy will be respected, that confidentiality will be preserved, that their identity will not
be disclosed without permission to others, researchers or

anyone else. Subjects consent to being in experiments on
the assumption that these conditions will be met. This means
that the researcher--any researcher, whether in medicine, in
the social sciences, or elsewhere--has a contractual obligation to respect the terms under which subject participation
is secured.

If the right to privacy means, roughly, the right to
control access of others to oneself, either through information about oneself or getting access to one's person, and if
confidentiality has something to do with the right to keep
information about oneself secret and non-public (Caplan,
1981), then the researcher in this case or in any case acts
unethically if he or she violates the terms of the experimental relationship. That is, there exists a contract with
certain conditions laid out; when those conditions are violated, then the violator has done something wrong. By simply disclosing the HLA type of a potential donor, the researcher (Krieger, in this case) violates privacy and confidentiality. The disclosure also opens the subject to
potential embarrassment, humiliation, and stress. One
might well find it hard to turn down a request to save somebody else's life knowing you're the only person that can do
it.

Most importantly, this kind of disclosure and related
cavalier transfers of information pose grave risks to the
entire research enterprise. Not only are certain prima
facie rights violated by that conduct, but the entire legal
apparatus that supports the research with human subjects in
the United States is undercut. When people are permitted
to chisel away at the body of law and contract governing
human experimentation, when persons begin to think they can
no longer trust the researcher to keep confidentiality or
to protect privacy, then pretty soon there will not be any
subjects to protect because no one will participate in
research.

There are in fact two types of moral wrongs that make
the conduct of exchanging information--in this case, even
to save a life--unethical. First, there is a violation of
binding promises and contracts. Second, and more importantly,
disclosure undercuts the entire moral and legal basis upon
which human experimentation and human research now proceed--
the contract between the researcher and the subject. I think
we have to be very careful about tolerating such conduct.

B. The Doctor/Patient Relationship

The doctor/patient relationship is both a fiduciary and contractual one, as is the nurse/patient relationship and the social worker/patient relationship. There exists a set of relationships between patients and health care professionals, not always explicit, but negotiated in subtle ways and subtle forms. Usually there is a statement by the patient of what he or she wants, the health professional listens, makes some judgment about whether he or she can go along with the request, and some sort of agreement is reached (Siegler, 1981). This process of negotiation of the terms and boundaries of the medical relationship is at the heart of the doctor/patient relationship.

It is interesting to note that in this case one might say that the little girl's doctor is trying to advance the best interests of her patient. She realizes that her patient needs bone marrow and sets about getting it. In one sense, I think she acts correctly. What most people want from their health care professional--be it a nurse, a physician, or a social worker--is that this person aggressively pursue their best interest (Beauchamp and Childress, 1979).

The problem in this case is that the physician, Dr. Robb, should know that there are problems with her obligation to advance her patient's self-interest. The primary problem is that the potential donor also needs some kind of protection of interests. When a physician is working to advance someone else's self-interest, the immediate concern is, can that physician work for two masters? By going to the potential donor, Mr. Plantar, and saying 'you are the only person that can donate,' the doctor in this case is putting herself in a position whereby she must serve the interests of two people rather than one. Plantar, the man who is the potential source of the needed tissue, has no protection of his interests. He does not have an agent to speak for him; he doesn't have anyone playing the equivalent physician role which Dr. Robb is playing for her patient. Dr. Robb is trying to juggle the best interests of the little girl against the best interests of Mr. Plantar. But that may not be possible for a single physician to do.

Perhaps the optimal thing to have done in this case in recruiting a donor is to find out if Mr. Plantar has a doctor. Why do I say that? Think about some very real

possibilities. What if Mr. Plantar is a psychotic? What
if he is suicidal? What if he is a paranoid? What if he
is dying? What if he has leukemia himself? What if he
needs a kidney? What if he says, 'I'll give bone marrow to
the little girl if she will give me a kidney?' The point is
that there are all kinds of conditions under which it would
be dubious to recruit Mr. Plantar. What we require in such
recruitment situations is an agent or a person who can protect the best interest of the donor. So what should have
happened in the case is once the information as to compatible
donors became available, then Dr. Robb should have en-
deavored to get in touch with Plantar's physician. There
should be a screening process in such cases. Physicians
who try to maximize everybody's self-interest simultaneously
will have a hard time of it. So that is why the conduct is
morally suspect in this case.

C. The Doctor/Society Relationship

The question does arise in this case as to whether we
might waive some of the promises and violate some interests
just a little bit, because there is a little girl's life on
the line. After all, there is an identified individual who
could really benefit from the gift of bone marrow tissue.
One might argue that Dr. Robb has an obligation to try and
do what she can to advance the interests of that little girl.
In fact some might say, it is really the doctor's obligation
not only to look after a patient but also to look out for
the best interests of society. And it might be argued that
the doctor/society relationship provides grounds for overriding some of the arguments that I have made concerning why
it is wrong to use available information to get in touch
with possible organ donors or to violate the terms of a
contract concerning this information.

It is possible to locate cases where this happens. For
example, the public health service tries to find people who
have venereal disease. Physicians have obligations to report
persons suffering from gunshot wounds to public authorities.
Similar laws govern spouse and child abuse. Is the protection of privacy to override the public interest?

I think there are moral grounds for overriding promises
and undercutting some of the terms of the doctor/patient
relationship and the subject/researcher relationship, but I
think they are not relevant to this case. The conditions

under which a physician is justified in laying aside responsibility to a patient's self-interest are in fact very narrow. The conditions that permit overriding personal interest in cases of gunshot wounds, venereal disease, reporting an epileptic, and so on are instances of real and significant danger. Moreover, it is potential danger to many that overrides the doctor/patient relationship, not the potential danger posed to a single person. The degree of certainty of danger serious to large numbers is what licenses physicians to act in the public interest.

The existence of promises, contracts, and special relationships do make a difference, because public health officials do not work for a patient. They work for the state, and they are agents of the state. They are hired to look out for the public interest and thus they are not useful examples for describing normal doctor/patient relationships and the ethics of these relations.

The arguments that have been made thus far concerning recruitment and disclosure reveal an acceptance of present conditions and present understandings of what the doctor/patient relationship is, what the subject/experimenter relationship is, and what the role is of the private physician relative to patient interests. However, one might ask, is that the way matters should be? I do not want to pursue that question, but surely the question is worth discussing. Much of my analysis presumes many things to be true or accepted about what we want our doctors to do, but I am not arguing that that is the way it has to be. Surely it is possible to argue that physicians should not pursue the interests of their patient. Perhaps it is possible to imagine a system in which they try to pursue simultaneously the gross or total interests of all the patients they come in contact with. Such a system might lead to different decisions about the behavior undertaken in this case, but it would not reflect current models of doctor/patient interaction in America today.

II. ETHICAL ISSUES IN ORGAN AND TISSUE DONATION

Who are the potential donors in any organ or tissue situation? The best candidates are living relatives. We already know there was one in the case under examination who said no. Then there are living strangers. Within this category there are doctors, there are health personnel, and there are medical students. They all have a sworn duty to save life. Maybe they are the first pool to approach after relatives. What other kinds of strangers are there? There are children, there are mentally incompetent people, there are ill people, there are prisoners, there are ordinary average adults, and there are elderly people. There is a whole range of possible candidates that one might want to canvass. Few of these people appear in the research proto- col that was done by the research physician in our case, but they all are potential donors. They are potential people who might be candidates--pooled, typed, registered, and so on. Who else is available? Near-dead strangers might be available; those most famous examples from ethics case studies and television shows, those on respirators and the near-brain-dead. There is small sample of such persons that could serve as donors (Childress, 1979). Then there are the newly dead; that is, those that we are sure are dead, but might still have some useful parts. Thus, there is a wide variety of potential donors.

A central problem with our case study is that no attention is given to many sources of supply. The physi- cians find themselves with a list of people who happened to be available and they attempt to list what they can. But, being on a list is hardly an argument for preferring live donors to dead ones.

Another key issue that deserves mention that is not discussed in the case, but that is morally relevant and affects the assessment of what is done, is possible modes of getting a supply of tissue. There are at least four ways to encourage the supply of organs and tissues.

One is voluntary donation by people who come forward and say, I want to give, I want to help, put my name on a list. That is the British system of blood donation, Richard Titmuss wrote about in his book The Gift Relationship (1971), and it is the system that as far as I know still prevails in Britain today with regard to blood supply. There are no commercial blood banks in England. Persons receive blood from those people who want to give it.

Another way to obtain organs or tissue is to allow people to sell them (Brams, 1977). This can be done by all the sources mentioned previously--from the nearly dead, from the newly dead, from strangers, or relatives. We might say put all organs up for bid. If a little girl wants an organ, let her purchase it from someone who wants to sell. Maybe more organs would become available that way.

Another possible way to obtain tissue is to have a draft. We could institute a conscription of tissues and organs when a person had died or was nearly dead. We would allow the state to take whatever parts are needed (Dukeminier and Sanders, 1968). The burden of protest in such a system would be put on those who want out of the system. If there is a person who for some reason objects, then it is their problem to get themselves out of the system. Other things being equal, society will take what is needed.

Finally, we could institute a policy of mandatory choice. That's the system represented in my wallet by a kidney card. The card does not say that anybody can take my kidney. Rather, it does make me decide one way or the other whether I want to be a donor. The card serves to encourage me to make a choice about donation, and, in fact, there are advertisements and other sorts of subtle pressure to get me to try to make a choice in favor of donation. Such cards do not entitle the state to take what it wants or the medical profession to have what it needs. A card system simply encourages individuals to think about making a donation.

These sources of supply are important, even though they don't come up in the case. But they are relevant to any organ or tissue donation question. The ethics of donation is contingent upon the ethics of the mode of supply.

What does it mean to have a full and complete voluntary donation? I think a voluntary donation occurs when full, free, informed consent is given. Happily, full and informed consent is the guiding norm governing human experimentation. Thus, there is no shortage of literature on the topic (Barber, 1980). What then is involved in full, informed consent? First, an effort must be made to determine competency to decide. We don't know what Plantar's competency is in this case. We don't know if he's crazy, we don't know if he is sick, we don't know what his story is. So, the competency question remains open as far as the case goes.

The second element of consent is freedom of choice. Minimally this requires the absence of coercion. What kinds

of things can be coercive? Among the factors contributing
to coercion are fear, the power of authority, embarrassment,
suddenness, and surprise can all be coercive. Having to
deal with someone who is explicitly identified to you can
be a very coercive thing to deal with. Economists know
that very well. We spend a lot more money to save identified lives than we do to save unidentified lives. We spend
a lot more money, for example, on renal dialysis than we do
per person on highway safety because we know exactly who
has renal failure. But we don't know, except statistically,
who the car accident victim is. Economic coercion is another form of coercion--for example, the incentive of free
care. Some people may think that if they donate tissue,
they might get free care in the hospital. Some people think
that public admiration may come to them--they can write
books or appear on the Johnny Carson show. Many people may
hope for the benefit of reciprocity--I'll give to you if
you'll give to me later. And those are forces which can be
coercive, especially on someone who might be sick or ill in
some way that is not explicitly discussed in the case.

Free choice and consent also imply knowledge. This is
the third element of consent. Does a person have knowledge
to base a decision upon? What is sufficient knowledge?
Full and complete disclosure of reasonable risks and benefits, disclosure of possible alternative sources for getting
the tissue and comprehension of the information would seem
necessary. In our case, it is said that Plantar is given
the opportunity to ask questions. I don't think that is a
reliable test of comprehension. In the case it is said
that Plantar is not told there is another relative who said
no; this fact is not disclosed. This behavior would seem
to violate the criteria for consent--is there sufficient
disclosure of things that reasonable people would want to
know? It is hard to believe that any reasonable person
wouldn't want to know about the existence of another possible donor. Moreover, it is impossible to believe that anybody wouldn't want to know about the fact that the only
source of potential donors that has been searched is the
list supplied by Dr. Krieger. So, all of these actions
cloud the moral picture that we have of the consent in this
case and of the terms under which consent was given. Ultimately, the case is morally troubling, specifically with
regard to the issue of consent. There is incomplete disclosure about information about matters such as what does
it mean to go into the hospital and lose a week's pay? Even

if it doesn't hurt to have bone marrow taken out, a person may not want to spend a week in the hospital (if that's what it takes). Who will compensate the donor if something does go wrong? This is not presented, but since such disclosure is a standard part of presentations in the human experimentation area, it should be here, too. Coming at someone out of the blue and saying, "Look, you've got to save X"--that's coercive, in my opinion. What is needed, certainly, is some kind of protection--that's why it was important for Dr. Robb to go to the other physician, Plantar's physician first, if he or she existed. If not, then I think it is important that the physicians locate someone to help Plantar make his decision. A physician seeking a donor must find out information about whether or not a donor is even approachable. So, there are many moral problems in the case about the way in which the approach and the so-called consent issues were conducted. There is no question that things were not done as well as they should be, ethically speaking.

III. MINIMAL CONDITIONS FOR ORGAN AND TISSUE DONATION

What should happen in voluntary organ donation that would meet ethically minimal requirements? If voluntary donation is the mode to supply, then:

(1) Recruitment of donors always must be done by those with no direct interest in the outcome.

(2) Recruitment should proceed when possible through physician-physician contact.

(3) Potential donors should be drawn by recruiters from a pool of persons who give consent in advance to be asked.

(4) Full disclosure of all information a la the standards of human experimentation must prevail in the consent process. Doctors have an obligation to inform to the same degree that they do when they are recruiting in the subject/experimenter relationship--they must disclose all reasonably relevant facts.

(5) Independent medical advice and counsel must be made available to prospective consenting donors.

(6) There should be a reasonable cooling-off period given to potential donors for decision making.

(7) Existing obligations and duties must be honored by all involved physicians towards all parties unless explicit consent is given to waive these.

(8) There ought to be a review body to make sure the procedures are honored.

REFERENCES

Barber B (1980). "Informed Consent in Medical Therapy and Research." New Brunswick: Rutgers University Press.

Beauchamp T, Childress J (1979). "Principles of Biomedical Ethics." New York: Oxford.

Brams M (1977). Transplantable human organs: should their sale be authorized by state statutes? Am Jrnl Law Med 3:183.

Caplan A (1981). The primacy of privacy. In Beauchamp TL, Faden R (eds): "Ethical Issues in Social Science Research," Baltimore: Johns Hopkins University Press, p 55.

Capron A (1974). Informed consent in catastrophic disease and treatment. Univ Penn Law Rev 123:364.

Childress J (1978). Rationing of medical treatment. In Reich W (ed): "Encyclopedia of Bioethics," New York: The Free Press, p 1414.

Dukeminier J, Sanders D (1968). Organ transplantation: a proposal for routine salvaging of cadaver organs. N Engl J Med 279:413.

Siegler M (1981). The doctor-patient encounter and its relationship to theories of health and disease. In Caplan A, Engelhardt HT, McCartney J (eds): "Concepts of Health and Disease," Reading: Addison-Wesley, p 627.

Titmuss RM (1971). "The Gift Relationship." New York: Pantheon.

Troubling Problems in Medical Ethics: The Third
Volume in a Series on Ethics, Humanism, and Medicine: 257–268
© **1981 Alan R. Liss, Inc., 150 Fifth Ave., New York, NY 10011**

THE RIGHT TO PRIVACY WHEN LIVES ARE AT STAKE

Gerald D. Abrams, M.D.

Department of Pathology
The University of Michigan
Ann Arbor, Michigan

INTRODUCTION

The case about to be considered raises a number of
specific issues in an area of fundamental importance to the
health care professions, the area of privacy and confidentiality. Since privacy and confidentiality are so vital
to the health professions, it would be well to explore some
of the broader aspects of such issues before focusing on
the finer details of the case.

At the outset, it would be fair to inquire what
interest a pathologist dealing with samples of blood, fluids,
exudates, and tissues derived from patients, might conceivably have in issues of privacy and confidentiality. The
answer, of course, has to do with storage and dissemination
of information. It takes but a moment's reflection to
realize that there is a greater concentration of highly
sensitive material in patients' medical records (and
associated hospital data banks) than almost anywhere else
in our culture. A significant fraction of this information
is generated nowadays in clinical laboratories under the
aegis of pathologists. Thus, inevitably, my colleagues and
I find ourselves to be curators of vast amounts of personal
data. I can assure you from my own experience that large
numbers of people are constantly after this information,
most of them properly so, some perhaps not.

The ethical problems generated by these conditions
are not new. Health care professionals, in fact, have been
concerned for centuries about dealing with sensitive

personal data entrusted to them. The problems have, however, been rendered more urgent these days by the virtually
effortless and instantaneous manipulation, processing, and
retrieval of data accomplished by electronic means. Any of
you who remember hunting for, and then rummaging through
barely legible hospital charts and records, and who are now
able to order up endless, neatly lettered lists on a CRT
just by touching a keyboard, are keenly aware of the urgency
and potential difficulties to which I allude.

THE NATURE AND IMPORTANCE OF PRIVACY

Most of you would probably accept, as a starting
position, that regard for the rights of the individual is a
guiding ethical principle of prime importance. This
principle is mirrored in the language of judicial opinions
(quoted by Meisel and Roth, 1978) handed down through the
years. Judge Flaherty, in a recent trial having to do with
bone marrow transplantation asserted that "Our society...
has as its first principle, the respect for the individual,
and that society and government exist to protect the
individual from being invaded and hurt by another". This
parallels Justice Cardozo's classical assertion that "Every
human being of adult years and sound mind has a right to
determine what shall be done with his body". It can be
argued, I believe, that information pertaining to one's
body and what goes on within it is but a slight extension
of the individual; and thus is entitled to the same sort
of consideration. That is to say, privacy and personal
integrity are inextricably intertwined.

Privacy involves many things, beginning with freedom
from unwanted intrusion of other people, sights, or sounds.
Another important aspect of privacy is being allowed to conduct certain activities in a solitary fashion, if desired;
and another is protection from disclosure of material
considered by the subject to be embarrassing.(Greenawalt,
1978) A vital part of this last aspect of privacy is
control over the dissemination of existing personal information about one's self. (Fried, 1968). Confidentiality is
an aspect of privacy which allows us to share sensitive
information with selected associates in a manner which preserves our feelings of privacy and sense of personal
integrity. (Winslade, 1978) Confidentiality is based on a
sort of contract which assures the individual about control,

i.e., volunteered information will be allowed to go
absolutely no further than the specified recipient. Arrangements involving privacy and confidentiality are literally
what allow us to live together, and at the same time
exchange intimacies and preserve a large degree of autonomy.

In the health care arena, privacy and confidentiality,
and the firm belief that they will be maintained, are
absolutely essential. Accurate diagnosis and selection of
appropriate therapy are utterly dependent upon the flow of
information. To obtain optimal care, a person must reveal
the most sensitive and personal matters without restraint,
secure in the guarantee that the proffered information will
go no further than the health care team; and by extension,
that the information will be used only in the diagnostic
and therapeutic process.

A corollary to these considerations of privacy and confidentiality is that the concerned individual is the only
one who can properly decide what is sensitive and private
in the mass of accumulated medical information. Predictably,
most people in our culture would be quite protective about
information relating to their sexual function. However, a
few others might be equally sensitive, with equal validity,
about their fasting blood sugar or history of tuberculosis.
It follows from this, that all medical data must be treated
as confidential. It would be inappropriate for those of us
who are curators of data banks to decide, on behalf of the
involved subjects, which data are sensitive and therefore
to be held confidential, and which are trivial and therefore eligible for dissemination.

POTENTIAL CONFLICT BETWEEN PRIVACY RIGHTS AND SOCIETAL NEEDS

Considerations such as those outlined above lead
easily to the construction of a neat ethical package in
which is embodied the notion that people are entitled to the
expectation of absolute privacy and confidentiality in
medical matters. Part of this expectation is that all
personal data will be used for absolutely no other purposes
than those for which the information was divulged, i.e.,
diagnosis and therapy. In the real world, however, matters
aren't so simple, and there are frequent collisions between
personal rights and societal needs. The fact of the matter
is that medical information is rather widely shared,

traveling well beyond the bounds imagined by most patients.
To be sure, most curators of medical information indulge in
sort of a triage process, deciding that some medical data
are worthy of more confidential treatment than others.
Embodied in this triage is an intuitive belief that the
patient's serum sodium concentration is less worthy of protection than his or her sexual history. By the same line
of reasoning, in many institutions, psychiatric records are
held separately (and tightly closed) from the rest of the
medical record; while in those same institutions it is
possible, at dozens of computer terminals, to retrieve data
about patients' blood chemistries, microbiological cultures,
and tissue biopsies. While most of us would approve these
sorts of arrangements in a general way, pointing to some
cost/benefit ratio in each instance, the system is difficult
to defend if one accepts the principle that only the
individual concerned can decide what is sensitive and what
is trivial in his or her record.

As one inspects the day-to-day operation of our health
care system, several different categories of data collection
and usage can be identified. Westin (1980) has described
three zones in which personal health data are collected.
Zone 1 is the zone of primary health care, a zone in which
medical information is obtained and used for direct diagnosis and treatment of the subject. Zone 2 involves the use
of medical information for administrative purposes in such
matters as payment for the services, and quality-of-care
reviews. Zone 3 encompasses the social uses of health data,
that is the uses which are quite separate from diagnosis and
treatment of the patient's problems; and in fact, which are
sometimes in conflict with the patient's own interests.

At first inspection, activities within Westin's Zone 1
would seem to pose very little ethical difficulty, and that
is generally so. Patients are likely to be aware that information they offer to the examining physician may be shared
amongst other members of the health care team. One readily
accepts this sort of sharing as necessary to the diagnostic
and therapeutic process. In large contemporary hospitals,
however, the practical requirements of moving data between
various members of the health care team are such that safeguards to privacy are not absolute. In other words, for the
attending physician to obtain certain laboratory data
expeditiously, it's generally necessary to transmit this
information to a variety of less-than-perfectly protected

terminals, or to transmit the information over the telephone when positive identification of the recipient is difficult. Furthermore, built into our major teaching hospitals is another bit of an ethical dilemma. Only a fraction of the information being passed around within such hospitals is for the benefit of the individual patients who yielded that information. Much of the information is used, instead, for purposes of educating the next generation of health care professionals. While training medical or nursing students may be a laudable goal, it undeniably involves sharing sensitive medical information for other than diagnostic and therapeutic reasons. Traditionally we deny the existence of an ethical dilemma in this sort of information-use by asserting that there is an element of implied consent involved when a patient enters what he or she knows to be a teaching hospital. It would seem more reasonable to strive wherever possible in the medical educational arena to obtain such consent in explicit rather than implicit terms.

With regard to information usage in Zone 2, patients generally recognize that it is necessary to divulge certain data in order that payers may review eligibility and assess claims. The importance of quality review is certainly also recognized. However, there exists in this zone a definite potential for abuse if there is not constant vigilance with regard to how much personal information really needs to be divulged for these administrative purposes, and what guarantees are extracted from the administrative recipients of that information as to how it will be protected.

The dissemination of medical information within Zone 3 is certainly the most troublesome potentially. In this area information is used, not for the good of the individual, but for what is deemed to be a larger good. Such uses include employment screening, licensing requirements, insurance, medical and social research, public health purposes, and even judicial or law enforcement purposes. There exists in this zone a spectrum of situations, from those rather clearly demanding some encroachment on individual rights for the good of the order, to those which are controversial to say the least. Most of us, when we board a commercial aircraft, would sincerely hope that the pilot has not been allowed to keep private something like the existence of a poorly controlled seizure disorder. Similarly, those of us who work in emergency rooms or morgues recognize the societal importance of reporting

gunshot wounds. Most reasonable people would also recognize
that if there is an epidemic of staphylococcal infection
ravaging the newborn nursery, it would be reasonable to
insist that nursery personnel submit to appropriate bacterio-
logic probing meant to detect the carrier state, irrespective
of their personal feelings. The problem becomes somewhat
more difficult when we consider the dilemma of a psychiatrist
whose patient threatens to break the law or to harm another
individual. A similar dilemma confronts the physician who
recognizes that his patient is having transient ischemic
attacks, but is told by that patient that he insists on
continuing his sole livelihood as a long distance truck
driver.

One could possibly justify each of the above examples
(albeit with some difficulty in the last two) on the grounds
that individual rights to privacy and confidentiality are
being encroached upon in order to prevent or alleviate an
imminent threat to some other individual or individuals.
There are, however, many other examples which could be drawn
in which Zone 3 uses of confidential information do not prevent some predictable harm from befalling persons other than
the subject. Rather, they are proposed on the grounds that
by disseminating the data, some persons other than the subject might conceivably be aided. The case about to be considered embodies one variation of this theme. In our medical
centers, a much more common Zone 3 phenomenon of this sort
is the use of medical information obtained in the diagnostic/
therapeutic setting for research purposes.

Obviously, a lot of this goes on, and often one can
point to concrete societal gains derived from the activity.
In much of the research done with medical information, we
employ, as outlined above, a sort of intuitive triage
system wherein the decision is made that the information to
be disseminated is trivial or neutral enough to be shared
beyond the circle of the subjects' physicians with little
concern. Thus, few people would be very excited about a
proposed chart review of our last fifty patients found to
have an elevated blood calcium, in order to determine the
ultimate fate of such patients. Similarly, most of us would
be fairly relaxed about a retrospective record-review of the
past ten year's experience with ovarian cancer. The argument
could be made that a) the data are not used in a name-linked
way once the information is extracted from charts; b) only
members of the health-care establishment are involved; and

(perhaps) c) implied consent for this sort of study is part of coming to a teaching hospital.

Problems in this area can, however, be much more difficult to resolve. Several days ago, I exchanged views about privacy and confidentiality with a group of our Pathology house officers in preparation for this conference. In the context of our discussion, the house officers agreed unanimously that they were ethically bound to prevent dissemination of data gathered in the diagnostic setting and entrusted to them. Literally ten minutes after our conference was over, a call came in to our Clinical Immunology Laboratory from a University physician who requested the names of the last twenty individuals found by the laboratory to have positive tests for syphilis on samples of their cerebrospinal fluid. The caller stated that he wished to have this information so that he could follow up with a study of the biological significance of such findings in the modern era. Immediately, the previously developed house officer consensus fell apart, with some individuals asserting that to divulge the information was perfectly all right since it was another physician requesting it; and with others equally vigorously claiming the duty to keep such sensitive information about a venereal disease strictly confidential. Many of the individuals arguing for confidentiality, however, stated that they would have been perfectly willing to yield a list of names had the request been for patients having an abnormality of some serum protein, for example. This view, of course, does not take into account the principle that only the subject himself or herself can decide what information is worthy of being held in confidence. Those individuals who thought it correct to share even sensitive information as long as it was within the health-care "family", and as long as it was for altruistic purposes, had difficulty maintaining that stand in slightly different circumstances. They had difficulty when I asked them if it would be proper to release to a sociologist the names of 50 men coming in with the complaint of impotence, for the purpose of studying the effect of sexual dysfunction on the fabric of family life.

Obviously these sorts of cases pose extremely difficult problems. Historically we have dealt with the problems rather informally, substituting our benevolent judgement for that of the patients who "own" the data in question; and implicitly arguing that a trivial encroachment upon privacy rights is justified by the ends to be served. However, moral judgements should differ in various cases only if morally relevant aspects of the cases in question differ. Therefore, articulating a moral principle which would allow violation of privacy in certain of the above situations but not in others would appear to be an impossible task.

VIOLATION OF PRIVACY RIGHTS. CONSEQUENCES AND SOLUTIONS

Whenever we consider overriding patients' absolute right to privacy and confidentiality we must squarely face the possible consequences, at both an individual and a societal level. Our traditional system of informal triage seems to me to be focused largely at the individual level, with care being taken not to harm individual subjects. To a large extent this approach appears to work, at least judged by the fact that we don't often get into trouble. However, in the long run, I believe we in the healing pro-fessions and society at large stand to lose a great deal by the gradual erosion of privacy rights. If our patients' expectations of privacy and confidentiality in dealing with us are shaken, there will inevitably be a chilling effect on the free exchange of information so necessary to optimal health care. This, of course, has been recognized for thousands of years, and indeed was embodied in the Hippocratic Oath.

In my view, the resolution of these difficult ethical problems involves prevention; i.e., we must pay much more attention than we customarily have to the a priori establish-ment of ground rules for obtaining and manipulating sensitive data. At the outset there should be explicit understandings with the patients as to the purposes for which the informa-tion they offer may be used. This would seem to be especially important in our teaching-center settings. There should be a specific prior understanding about release of information for any but immediate health care purposes. We must also evolve explicit organizational policies about handling of stored data. (Steele, 1980) Persons involved in handling medical data must be highly trained in the legal and ethical aspects of their jobs. Access to data must be controlled on some reasonable need-to-know basis. The en-tire data handling system must be surveyed constantly by some "watchdog" mechanism to correct potential abuses. If and when our data handling can be described in this fashion,

it should be possible to take maximal advantage of contemporary technology, not only in the up-grading of medical
care but also in the service of broader societal aims,
without threatening the right to privacy so important to
our patients.

THE CASE

The case presented to us for discussion is an excellent
vehicle for bringing issues about privacy into focus. The
case is dramatically drawn in that it pits the privacy rights
of one individual against a chance to save the life of
another. However, the ethical issues involved are those
discussed above more generally in the consideration of
Zone 3 uses of medical information (i.e., the encroachment
upon one's privacy rights to serve a purpose unrelated to
that individual).

The case would be an excellent one if only to prompt
discussion of hypothetical ethical issues; but there is
also a genuine immediacy to it. Transplantation of bone
marrow from a donor to an unrelated recipient is not a
futuristic dream, it has already been accomplished.
(Westminster Hospitals Bone Marrow Transplant Team, 1977;
O'Reilly et al, 1977; Steinbrook, 1980)   That is, bone
marrow donors have been selected from large panels of HLA
typed individuals. A survey of the appropriate medical
literature suggests that bone marrow, in fact, is close to
joining corneas and kidneys in the routine repertoire of
the transplant team. Another fact which lends immediacy to
the case is that large scale programs are now being considered (Wieckowicz, 1975) in which HLA typed individuals
would be identified as prospective donors for matched blood
platelet transfusion. When one realizes that HLA typing
is also the key to kidney transplantation as well as to
bone marrow transplantation, the possible impact of HLA information becomes clear. I believe that even those individuals who are willing to attempt benevolent triage of data
in making ethical decisions would identify a person's HLA
type as something highly significant and worthy of privacy
protection.

One can only hope that the many thorny ethical issues
associated with tissue typing will be properly addressed
before such programs are activated. At very least, the

implications of HLA typing should be explained to individuals thinking of joining various sorts of donor panels. There needs to be explicit a priori permission relating to specific uses of HLA data (e.g., can information obtained for the platelet transfusion program be released to bone marrow or renal transplant teams?). In a sense, the need for these safeguards is particularly acute in the case of donor panels for various blood products, since individuals who identify themselves for such purposes are clearly more altruistic than the general population and therefore, are potentially more susceptible to undue pressure applied to them in other settings. Another, unrelated but interesting ethical issue revolves about the fact that persons with some HLA types are susceptible to certain serious diseases, which cannot now be prevented. Should such information be shared with the subjects by the directors of the donor operation?

The case at hand actually embodies two sorts of privacy issues. The first has to do with the proper control over HLA haplotype information gained in an experimental setting. This particular issue in my opinion would be the same whether just one doctor was involved instead of two, as indicated in the protocol. In other words, Brian Plantar volunteered as a subject in a medical research project, and presumably signed a consent form which delineated the type of information sought and the uses to which it would be put. The right to privacy and confidentiality in this situation would appear to be precisely parallel to that inherent in the health care situation, i.e., there is a sort of contract which circumscribes the use of information. Given the character of HLA data, as outlined above, this is clearly sensitive information. One might argue that Mr. Plantar loses relatively little in this case when his privacy is violated by his being approached as a donor, compared to what is potentially to be gained by the bone marrow recipient. However, just as in the case of "ethical triage" in a health care setting, the larger issue must be addressed. We must consider the extent to which there would be a chilling effect on medical research volunteers if privacy and confidentiality were not rigidly protected. Such a chilling effect, when considered in a total societal perspective, might be deemed to outweigh the possible (not guaranteed) benefit to a single individual.

If one were to conclude that breach of privacy is not permissible in the manner outlined in the case, one might

seek creative solutions, given the existence of the information about Plantar. One solution which suggests itself is
to send a form letter to each of the members of the HLA
typed panel asking them to reply if they would consider
becoming bone marrow donors. Even if there were sufficient
time to allow the use of this mechanism, one would have to
consider the ethical aspects of even using a mailing list
derived from the experimental panel. That is to say, one
might have to consider membership per se in the experimental
panel as confidential information, in which case the construction of a mailing list would be unethical. Another
possible approach would be to ask Plantar, directly, if he
had ever considered or would consider becoming a bone
marrow donor. This is subject to the same potential ethical
objection, in that confidentiality would have had to have been
breached simply to identify Plantar as a person to be
approached. In addition, at a more homely and practical
level, if Plantar were to respond to such an approach by
saying that he might consider being a bone marrow donor, it
would become quickly obvious to him that he had been "set-
up" when lo-and-behold, there just happened to be an
individual in dire need of his marrow. These ethical
difficulties highlight the need always to consider the potential uses of information before it is gathered and to
obtain appropriate explicit permission from those involved.

A second sort of privacy consideration in this case is
the manner of the approach ultimately made to Plantar. It
can be argued that one has a right to maintain complete
control over his or her decision to make a gift of some
body constituent. To the extent that such decision is
coerced, it is an assault on the autonomy and integrity of
the individual. Certainly, permission obtained under
coercive conditions is invalid. In the best of all possible
ethical worlds, maximum information should be supplied to a
prospective donor at a time of minimal emotional commitment
to a given case in order to keep coercion to a minimum.

I hope this rather general and global consideration of
privacy and confidentiality in the health care arena has
made you all a bit uncomfortable, but at the same time
has provided you with a framework within which to explore
your own views and other options relating to this most

interesting case.

REFERENCES

Fried C (1968). Privacy. Yale Law J 77:475.
Greenawalt K (1978). Privacy. In Reich WT (ed): "Encyclo-
    pedia of Bioethics," New York: Free Press, p 1356.
Meisel A, Roth LH (1978). Must a Man be his Cousin's Keeper?
    Hastings Cent Rep 8:5.
O Reilly RJ, Dupont B, Pahwa S, et al (1977). Reconstitution
    in Severe Combined Immunodeficiency by Transplantation of
    Marrow from an Unrelated Donor. N Eng J Med 297:1311.
Steele MC (1980). Medical Confidentiality - The Design Issue
    of the 80's. In "Proceedings, The Fourth Annual Symposium
    on Computer Applications in Medical Care," IEEE, p 381.
Steinbrook R (1980). Unrelated Volunteers as Bone Marrow
    Donors. Hastings Cent Rep 10:11.
Westin AF (1980). Privacy and Health Data Systems: Experiences
    of 1960-1980 and Projections for the 1980's. In
    Lindberg DAB, Kaihara, S (eds): "MEDINFO 80," North-Holland,
    p. 276.
Westminster Hospitals Bone-Marrow Transplant Team (1977).
    Bone Marrow Transplantation from an Unrelated Donor for
    Chronic Granulomatous Disease. Lancet:210.
Wieckowicz MB(1975). "Single Donor Platelet Transfusions"
    Scientific, Legal, and Ethical Considerations." Washington:
    DHEW Publication No.(NIH)76-1059.
Winslade WJ (1978). Confidentiality. In Reich WT (ed):
    "Encyclopedia of Bioethics," New York: Free Press, p 194.

Troubling Problems in Medical Ethics: The Third
Volume in a Series on Ethics, Humanism, and Medicine: 269-271
© **1981 Alan R. Liss, Inc., 150 Fifth Ave., New York, NY 10011**

DISCUSSION SUMMARY: THE RIGHT TO PRIVACY WHEN LIVES ARE AT
                      STAKE

Marc D. Basson
Director, CEHM
University of Michigan
Ann Arbor, Michigan

The discussants generally decided that the process by
which Mr. Plantar had been told of Evon's need for his
donation was deceitful (because of the failure to mention
Evon's aunt) and coercive by virtue of a deliberate attempt
to play on his sympathies. A few physicians in the groups
disagreed with at least the latter point. They suggested
that Evon's doctor ought to serve as her advocate and could
quite appropriately be histrionic so long as he was not
threatening, for the former was simply strong argument while
the latter would be coercive. It was then decided to put
this issue aside and to concentrate on the prior breach of
confidentiality by Dr. Krieger.

The participants were virtually unanimous in asserting
that it had been unethical for Dr. Krieger (the researcher)
to break the confidentiality of his study results. They
argued not only that Mr. Plantar had a prima facie right to
privacy extending to his HLA type but also that the researchers
had certainly guaranteed Plantar such confidentiality in
obtaining their initial informed consent from him. Krieger
therefore seemed doubly in the wrong and few were prepared
to accept his action even when Evon's life seemed at stake.

Participants in several groups suggested that to fail
to give Plantar the opportunity to save Evon might also be a
wrong since this would deny him the opportunity to perform a
morally praiseworthy act. Together with discussants' strong
sympathies for Evon, this motivated many attempts to devise
a plan by which Evon might be saved without wronging Plantar.
Versions of three controversial proposals ultimately emerged

in each group.

The first proposal was for Dr. Krieger to contact Plantar himself, explaining the situation and asking his permission to give Plantar's name and phone number to Evon's doctors. Many were dissatisfied with this since it still seemed to them to be subjecting Mr. Plantar to a highly stressful request without his permission. However, it ultimately was approved by about 50% of the discussants. This approval was motivated by the lack of better proposals as well as by the argument that a request such as this might be stressful but should not be taken as unduly coercive if properly phrased.

Almost 20% of the dicussants voted to have Krieger contact Mr. Plantar's personal physician and ask him to put the request to Plantar. They felt that this would be less stressful for Plantar since his own doctor would clearly seem to be "on Plantar's side" rather than having Evon's interests at heart. They also pointed out that Plantar might be medically unsuitable for the donation and that checking with his physician first would in this case save a good deal of embarrassment all around. Those opposing this option suggested that it was unwieldy and would waste precious time, that having Plantar's personal physician ask him might be even more coercive because Plantar probably knew and respected his doctor, and finally that contacting Plantar's physician without consent was in itself a major breach of confidentiality.

There was initially a good deal of support for a third option, that Plantar be contacted and asked if he would like his name handed over if it should ever turn out that he might be a suitable donor. It was felt that this would be non-coercive and involve no breach of confidentiality. However, support for this idea dwindled rapidly in the face of strong objections to the implicit deceit in such a request.

About one fourth of the participants ultimately rejected any attempt to contact Mr. Plantar because of the apparent impossibility of doing so without interfering with his privacy in some way. These discussants suggested such diverse alternatives as screening the hospital staff for potential donors, public appeals in the mass media for potential donors, and contacting other institutions who

might have already created a pool of willing donors. If
none of these plans discovered a willing and compatible
potential donor, then 25% were regretfully prepared to allow
Evon to die rather than breach Plantar's privacy. They
pointed out that even with the donation we could not be
certain Evon would live.

There was also discussion in several groups about the
appropriate moral evaluation of Dr. Robb (Evon's doctor) in
the case as described. Although most felt he was wrong to
use the information Dr. Krieger should not have given him,
about 15% of the participants approved of Dr. Robb's action.
They claimed that Dr. Robb could not be bound by Dr. Krieger's
agreement with Plantar. "It may have been wrong for Krieger
to give the information to Robb," summarized one medical
student, "but given that he did so, I do not believe Robb
did wrong in making use of it. Robb's prime obligation is
to Evon, his patient, and he should be prepared to do a
great deal to help her."

**Troubling Problems in Medical Ethics: The Third
Volume in a Series on Ethics, Humanism, and Medicine: 273–279
© 1981 Alan R. Liss, Inc., 150 Fifth Ave., New York, NY 10011**

REFERENCES

GENERAL

Basson MD (ed) (1980). "Ethics, Humanism, and Medicine."
New York: Alan R. Liss, Inc.
Basson MD (ed)(1981). "Rights and Responsibilities in
Modern Medicine." New York: Alan R. Liss, Inc.
Beauchamp TL, Childress JF (1979). "Principles of Bio-
medical Ethics." New York: Oxford University Press.
Beauchamp TL, Walters L (1978). "Contemporary Issues in
Bioethics." Belmont, California: Wadsworth Publishing
Company, Inc.
Gorovitz S, et al. (eds)(1976). "Moral Problems in Medicine."
New Jersey: Prentice-Hall.

SIXTH CONFERENCE

Affirmative Action in Medical School Admissions

Alevy v Downstate Medical Center of the State of New York,
39 NY 2d 326, 348 NE 3d 537, 384 NYS 2d 82 (1976).
Bakke v The Regents of the University of California, 18 Cal
3d 34, 553 P.2d 1152, 132 Cal Rptr 680 (1976), cert.
granted, 97 SCt1089 (1977).
Cohen C (1977). Race and the equal protection of the laws.
Lincoln Law Review 10(2):117.
DeFunis v Odegaard, 82 Wash. 2d 11,507 P.2d 1169 (1973).
Geiger HJ, Sidel VW (1978). Medical school admissions: The
case for quotas. Hastings Center Report 8(5):18.
Nagel T (1973). Equal treatment and compensatory discrim-
ination. Philosophy and Public Affairs 2:348.
Rawls J (1971). "A Theory of Justice." Cambridge,
Massachusetts: Harvard University Press.
Scarpelli DG (1975). Minority admissions -- a realistic
assessment. N Eng J Med 292(16):860.
Letters (1975). Minority Students. N Eng J Med 293(4):206.
Sowel T (1970). Colleges are skipping over competent blacks
to admit "authentic" ghetto types. New York Times
Magazine, December 13:36.

Drug Testing in Prisons

Ayd FJ (1972). Drug studies in prisoner volunteers. Southern Medical Journal 65:440.

Capron AM (1973). Medical research in prisons. Hastings Center Report 3(3):4.

Cardon PV, Dommel FW Jr, Trumble RR (1976). Inquiries to research subjects: A survey of investigators. N Eng J Med 295:650.

Freedman B (1975). A moral theory of informed consent. Hastings Center Report 5(4):32.

Freund P (ed)(1970). "Experimentation with Human Subjects." New York: George Braxiller.

Hatfield F (1977). Prison research: The view from inside. Hastings Center Report 7(1):11.

Hodges RE, Bean WB (1967). The use of prisoners for medical research. JAMA 202(Nov 6):177.

Levine RJ, Lebacqz K (1979). Ethical considerations in clinical trials. Clin Pharmacol Ther 25:728.

Levine RJ (1979). Clarifying the concepts of research ethics. Hastings Center Report 9(3):21.

Mitford J (1972). Experiments behind bars: Doctors, drug companies, and prisoners. In "Kind and Unusual Punishment." New York: Alfred Knopf, Inc. Reprinted in Gorovitz (ed)(1976). "Moral Problems in Medicine."

The National Commission for the Protection of Human Subjects of Biomedical and Behavioral Resarch (1976). "Appendix to Report and Recommendation: Research Involving Prisoners." DHEW Publication No. (OS)76-132. (Many excellent papers including "On Doing it for Money" by Marx Wartofsky).

Travitzky DE (1977). Volunteering at Vacaville. Hastings Center Report 7(1):13.

Zaraphonetis CJD, et al. (1978). Clinically significant adverse effects in a phase I testing program. Clin Pharmacol Ther 24(2):127.

Zimmerman D (1981). Coercive wage offers. Philosophy and Public Affairs 10:121.

Treating Children Without Parental Consent

Ackerman TF (1980). The limits of beneficence: Jehovah's
    Witnesses and childhood cancer. Hasting Center Report
    10(4):13.
Annas GJ (1979). Reconciling Quinlan and Saikewicz: Decision
    making for the terminally ill incompetent. Am J Law
    and Med 4:367.
Burt RA (1979). "Taking Care of Strangers: The Role of
    Law in Doctor-Patient Relations." New York: Free
    Press.
Custody of a Minor. Massachusetts, 379 N.E. 2d 1053. (The
    Chad Green Case).
Dworkin G (1972). Paternalism. The Monist 56:64.
Jones v Saikewicz, 1977 Adv Sh (SJC) 2461 (Nov 28, 1977).
Leake HC, Rachels J, Foot P (1979). Active euthanasia
    with parental consent. Hastings Center Report 9(5):19.
McLellan MF (1977). Jehovah's Witnesses and child protection
    legislation: The right to refuse medical consent.
    Legal Medical Quarterly 1(March):37.
Ramsey P (1978). The Saikewicz precedent: What's good
    for an incompetent patient? Hastings Center Report
    8(6):36.
Relman A (1978). The Saikewicz decision: Judges as physi-
    cians. N Eng J Med 298(March 2):508.
Letters (1978). The Saikewicz decision. N Eng J Med 298
    (May 25):1208.
Schowalton JE, Ferholt JB, Man NM (1973). The adolescent
    patient's decision to die. Pediatrics 51(Jan):97.
    Reprinted in Gorovitz (ed)(1976). "Moral Problems
    in Medicine."
Siegler M (1977). Critical illness: The limits of autonomy.
    Hastings Center Report 7(5):12.
Waldman AM (1976). Medical ethics and the hopelessly ill
    child. J Pediat 88:990.

The Decision to Resuscitate - Slowly

Benjamin M (1979). Moral agency and negative acts in
    medicine. In Pritchard and Robison (eds). "Medical
    Responsibility." Clifton, New Jersey: Humana Press,
    pp 169-180.
Brody DS (1980). The patient's role in clinical decision
    making. Ann Int Med 93:718.

Collins VJ (1968). Limits of medical responsibility in
     prolonging life. JAMA 206(Oct):389.
Dworkin G (1972). Paternalism. The Monist 56:64.
Foot P (1977). Euthanasia. Philosophy and Public Affairs
     6(Winter):85.
Leake HC, Rachels J, Foot P (1979). Active euthanasia
     with parental consent. Hastings Center Report 9(5):19.
Lo B, Jensen AR (1980). Clinical decisions to limit treat-
     ment. Ann Int Med 93:764.
Menzel P (1979). Are killing and letting die morally dif-
     ferent in medical contexts? J Med and Phil 4(Sept):269.
Rabkin MT, Gillerman G, Rice NR (1976). Orders not to re-
     suscitate. N Eng J Med 295(Aug 12):364.
Rachels J (1975). Active and passive euthanasia. N Eng J
     Med 292(Jan 9):78.
Rachels J (1980). Euthanasia. In Regan T (ed). "Matters
     of Life and Death." New York: Random House, pp 28-66.
Veatch RM (1976). "Death, Dying and the Biological Revolution."
     New Haven: Yale Press.

SEVENTH CONFERENCE

Competency and the Right to Refuse Treatment

Baumgarten E (1980). The concept of competence in medical
     ethics. J Med Ethics 6(5):180-184.
Brady BA, Englehardt HT (eds) (1980). "Mental Illness:
     Law and Public Policy." Boston: D Reidel.
Chayet NL (1976). Informed consent of the mentally dis-
     abled: A failing fiction. Psych Ann 6:82ff.
Guttheil TG, Appelbaum PS (1980). Substituted judgment and
     the physician's dilemma: With special reference to
     the problem of the psychiatric patient. J Clin Psych
     41:303.
Macklin R (1977). Consent, coercion, and conflicts of
     rights. Persp Biol Med 20:360.
Roth LH, Meisel A, Lidz CW (1977). Tests of competency
     to consent to treatment. Am J Psych 134:279.
Starkman MN, Youngs DD (1979). Evaluation and management
     of the patient who refuses medical care. Primary
     Care 6:451.

Stowers v Wolodzko 191NW 2d 355 (MI Sup Ct Nov. 9, 1971).
Szasz T (1974). "The Myth of Mental Illness". New York:
    Harper and Row.
Wear S (1980). Mental illness and moral status. J Med
    Phil 5:292.

When Doctor and Nurse Disagree

Aroskar MA (1980). Anatomy of an ethical dilemma. Am J
    Nursing 80:658.
Aroskar MA, Flaherty MJ, Smith JM (1977). The nurse and
    orders not to resuscitate. Hastings Center Report
    7(4):27.
Carpenter WT, Langsner CA (1975). The nurse's role in
    informed consent. Nursing Times 71:1049.
Cawley MA (1977). Euthanasia: Should it be a choice? Am
    J Nursing 77:859.
Churchill L (1977). Ethical issues of a profession in
    transition. Am J Nursing 77:873.
Davis AJ, Aroskar MA (1978). "Ethical Dilemmas and Nursing
    Practice." New York: Appleton-Century-Croft.
Hirshaut Y, Bleich D (1975). Choosing a therapy when doctors
    disagree. Hastings Center Report 5(2):19.
Hull RT (1980). Blowing the whistle while you work. Kansas
    Nurse 55(11):7.
Hull RT (1980). Models of nurse/patient/physician relations.
    Kansas Nurse 55(9):19.
Johnson P (1977). The gray areas - who decides? Am J
    Nursing 77:856.
Murphy CP (1978). The moral situation in nursing. Chapter
    13 in Bandman EL, Bandman B (eds)(1978). "Bioethics
    and Human Rights." Boston: Little Brown and Co.
Ross WS (1972). Clinical research is the best medicine.
    Medical Opinion (Feb):51.
Smith SJ, Davis, AJ (1980). Ethical dilemmas: Conflicts
    among rights, duties, and obligations. Am J Nursing
    80:1463.
Stein LI (1967). The doctor-nurse game. Arch Gen Psychiat
    16:699.

Doctor Draft: Redistributing Physicians

Bellen LE (1976). Quality and equality in health care --
    What can we do about it? In Gorcvitz S et al. (eds)
    (1976). "Moral Problems in Medicine." New Jersey:
    Prentice Hall.
Dellums RV (1978). "A bill to establish a United States
    Health Service." 95th Congress, 2nd session. HR 11879.
    Washington: Government Printing Office.
Dellums RV (1979). The health services act. Congressional
    Record 125 (35) March 19.
Green RL (1978). Urban health care: How deficient is it?
    National Forum (Spring):18.
Kleinig J (1976). Good samaritanism. Philosophy and Public
    Affairs 5(4):382.
Outka G (1974). Social justice and equal access to health
    care. J Religious Ethics 2(Spring):11.
Page BB (1975). Who owns the professions? Hastings Center
    Report 5(5):7.
Sade RM (1971). Madical care as a right: A refutation.
    N Eng J Med 285:1288.
Sedgwick P (1974). Medical individualism. Hastings Center
    Report 2(3):69.
Starr PA (1975). A national health program: Organizing
    diversity. Hastings Center Report 5(1):11.
Steiner H (1976). The just provision of health care: A
    reply to Elizabeth Telfer. J Med Ethics 2:185.
Szasz TS (1969). The right to health. Georgetown Law J
    57:734. Reprinted in Gorovitz et al. (eds)(1976). "Moral
    Problems in Medicine."
Telfer E (1976). Justice, welfare, and health care. J Med
    Ethics 2:107.

The Right to Privacy When Lives are at Stake

Fried C (1968). Privacy. Yale Law J 77:475.
Greenawalt K (1974). Privacy and its legal protections.
    Hastings Center Studies 2(3):45.
Greenawalt K (1978). Privacy. In "Encyclopedia of Bioethics."
    3:1356 New York: MacMillan Press.
Jameton JA, Dukeminier J (1978). Organ donation. In
    "Encyclopedia of Bioethics." 3:1152 New York: MacMillan
    Press.

Jonas H (1969). Philosophical reflections on experimenting with human subjects. New York, NY:The Daedalus Library, American Academy of Arts and Sciences.

Levine MD et al. (1975). The ethics of bone marrow trans plantation. J Pediatr 86:145.

Meisel A, Roth LH (1978). Must a man be his cousin's keeper? Hastings Center Report 8(5):5.

Rachels J (1975). Why privacy is important. Phil and Pub Aff 4:295.

Scanlon T (1975). Thomson on privacy. Phil and Pub Aff 4:315.

Schwitzgeld RB (1969). Confidentiality of research in public health studies. Harv Legal Comm 6:187.

Thomas ED (1978). Marrow transplantation for acute leukemia. Cancer 42(Suppl):895.

Thomas ED, Buckner CD, Clift RA, et al. (1979). Marrow transplantation for acute nonlymphoblastic leukemia in first remission. N Eng J Med 301:597.

Thomas ED, Storb R (1970). Technique for bone marrow grafting. Blood 36:507.

Thomson JJ (1975). The right to privacy. Phil and Pub Aff 4:295.

Westin AF (1976). "Computers, Health Records, and Citizen Rights." Washington, DC: US Dept of Commerce, National Bureau of Standards Monograph 157.

Index

ANA Code for Nurses, 179, 187, 191
Abortion, 147
Absolution, ethical, 146–148
Admission to medical school, 4, 9–48
Admissions criteria, 10, 34, 41
Adversarial due process (see also: court intervention), 102–108, 115–116
Affirmative action, 9–48
Altruism (See also: benificence), 86, 91, 266
Analysis, ethical (see also: moral language, meaning of), xv, 246
Arguments, ethical, xv, 145
Autonomy (see also: libertarianism), 5, 62, 70, 124–125, 160, 167, 211, 223, 258–259, 267

Bakke, 9–10, 20, 22–38
    benificence (see also: altruism; donation), 218, 225
    bias, 5, 104–105, 128, 152, 166

Children, 7, 95–116, 157, 163–164
Civil Rights Act, 10, 18, 20–22
Code/no code decisions, 117–118, 121, 133–134, 137, 139, 141
Coercion (see also: consent), 49–50, 63–67, 69, 80–81, 91, 217, 252–253, 267, 269–270
Committee on Ethics, Humanism and Medicine, xiv–xvii
Compensation, 9–10, 18–20
Competence, 4–7, 103, 124, 138 151–178, 252

case law examples, 162–164, 170, 172, 174–175
    criteria for, 162
    determination of, 172, 175–176
    kinds of, 152, 158–160
    of lawyers, 173–174
    practical guidelines for, 172–173
Confidentiality (see also: right to privacy), 258–259
Conflicts, 102, 166
Consent (see also: coercion)
    implied, 169, 263
    informed, 3–4, 62–65, 67–69, 80–81, 87–89, 96, 109–111, 118, 124, 137, 139, 165, 169, 245, 252–254
    presumed, 169
    proxy, 6, 95–116, 118, 122, 131, 134, 139, 161, 177
    vicarious, 169
Constitution, 10, 22–38, 208, 224
Contracts (see also: relationships), 247–248, 250, 258–259
Cost-benefit analysis (see also: scarcity of resources), 3, 72, 78, 118, 162, 240, 253
Court intervention (see also: adversarial due process; law, purpose of), 7, 85–86, 96, 99, 106–107, 111, 114, 131, 135, 138, 151–152, 161, 200
    justification for, 96, 103, 112
Davis program (see: Bakke)
Deceit, 118, 127, 142, 269–270
Decision to not resuscitate (see also: code/no code decisions), 117–141

Decision-making (see also: consent), 3–8, 16, 102, 131, 134–136, 138, 160–162

Dilemmas, ethical, 49–50, 57–62, 70–72, 179, 239–240, 261–262

Discrimination (see also: preference, reverse discrimination), 9, 18, 20–21, 24, 26, 63–64

Distribution of benefits, 9–10, 18, 218–221

Distribution of physicians (See also: redistribution of physicians), 207, 215–221, 227–232

Diversity of student body, 24–25, 27, 28–29

Doctor/nurse disagreements (see Doctor-nurse relationship)

Doctor-Nurse relationship, 179–206
  importance of communication, 181, 193
  reasons for disagreement, 194, 197–198
  resolution of disagreements, 201

Doctor-patient relationships, 193–194, 239, 246, 248–250, 264, 269
  fiduciary, 178
  how to talk with patients, 169–170
  resolution of disagreements, 201–202

Doctor-patient trust, 110, 135, 142, 195

Doctor-society relationship, 207–238, 249–250

Donation, organ (see also: benificence), 250–255, 265–267

Drug testing, 49–94

Economic considerations (see: Scarcity of resources)

Equal protection, 9–10, 17–18, 20–21, 25, 224

Equal treatment, 218–221

Error, ethical, 3, 7, 146, 148

Ethics, theories of (see also: Kant; moral language, meaning of; utilitarianism)

Euthanasia (see also: decision not to resuscitate; harm), 4, 6, 141
  active vs. passive, 126–127, 134

Experimentation (see: research)

Exploitation, 66, 70, 74

Fairness (see: Justice)

Family, 5–6, 95–96, 111, 138, 165, 250

God, 3, 4

Harm, 5, 49
  vs. failure to help (see also: euthanasia), 222

Health care, 4, 189–192

Helsinki, Declaration of, 63

ICU (See: Intensive Care Unit)

Idealism, ethical, 49–50, 57–62, 70–72

Inducements, 49–50, 54, 63–67, 73–75, 81–82, 92–93

Informed consent (See: Consent)

Insanity (See: competence)

Intensive Care Unit, 118, 119–122, 124–125, 132–133, 137–138, 187–189
  nursing experiences in, 187–188

Interests, 5–6

Intuition, moral, xv, 7, 146–147, 214

Involuntary commitment, 170–172

Jehovah's Witnesses, 157, 159, 162

Justice, 9, 18–19, 36, 49, 192, 223–224, 236

Kant, 49, 60–61, 211, 215–218

Knowledge, medical, 222–223

Law, purpose of (see also: court intervention; justification)

Lawyer-client relationship, 173–174

Legal vs. ethical obligations, 95, 166

Libertarianism, 49, 157, 208, 213–215

Living will (see also: Consent, proxy), 161

Logical ethics, xv, xvii, 145–149, 217

Lottery, 10, 47

Medical education
  benefits and obligations, 227–234
Merit, 10, 16, 47
Metaethics (see: moral language,
  meaning of)
Moral language, meaning of, 60–61,
  145–149

National health insurance, 207, 209–21C
Nazis, 4, 148
National Health Service, 207–211, 233
Need, 218–221
Nuremberg Code, 63, 65

Obligations, nursing (see also:
  relationships; rights; roles), 179,
  180
  to doctors, 185, 187
  to institutions, 185, 187, 203
  to oneself, 187
  to patients and their families, 185,
  187, 204, 248
  to the nursing profession, 187, 204
  to the state, 187
Orders, 4

Paternalism, 3, 5, 110, 116, 118, 140,
  188
Patient, 5
Pay scales (see: inducements)
Placebo, 6
Pluralism, ethical, 148–149
Preference (see also: discrimination),
  9, 17–23, 29–30
Principles, ethical, 146–147, 189
Prisoners, 49–94, 159
  living conditions of, 51–53

Quality of life (see also Intensive Care
  Unit), 199–200
Questions
  ethical, 166
  medical, 166
Quinlan, Karen Ann, 163, 200

Quotas, 10, 16, 23, 26–28, 31, 34, 47

Race, 9–48, 49, 64, 83–84
Reasonableness, 151
Redistribution of physicians, 207–238
Refusal of treatment (see also:
  consent), 6–7, 95–116, 151–178
Relationships (see: doctor-nurse;
  doctor-patient; doctor-society;
  lawyer-client; researcher-subject;
  obligations)
Relativism, ethical, 147–148
Research, 49–94, 214, 239, 246–247,
  262, 266
  review, 50
  therapeutic vs. non-therapeutic,
  76–77
Researcher-subject relationship,
  246–247, 249–250, 266
Reverse discrimination (see also:
  discrimination), 9, 32–33, 37
Rights
  Civil, 17–38, 62, 68
  human, 49–50, 57–59, 61–63, 68–69
  meaning of, 214
  of children, 102, 114
  of doctors, 208, 211, 237
  of individuals, 223–224, 258
  over children, 101
  to act foolishly, 5
  to decide, 49
  to health care, 232
  to know (see: truthtelling)
  to medical care, 190, 214, 219–221,
  222, 237
  to privacy, 145, 171, 239–272
  to refuse treatment (see also:
  refusal), 95–116, 123–124,
  170–171, 177
  to one's actions (see also:
  autonomy), 219–222, 258
Risks, 54–55, 64, 67–69, 75–76, 88–89,
  92, 242, 254
Roles (see also: relationship)
  doctor, 109, 179

nurse, 179, 195–196
university, 35–37

Scarcity of resources, 117–118, 122, 123, 126, 127–128, 141–142, 249–252
Senility, 7
Slow code (see also: code/no code decisions), 117, 131, 141
Socialized medicine, 207, 209
Society, interests of, 5, 9–10, 24, 37, 48, 49, 57–58, 68, 72, 91, 122, 162, 208, 259–262

Truthtelling, 95, 109–111, 121, 122, 124–125

Uncertainty, 3–8
Utilitarianism, 3, 49, 190, 218

Values, 5

PROGRESS IN CLINICAL AND BIOLOGICAL RESEARCH

Series Editors   Vincent P. Eijsvoogel   Seymour S. Kety
Nathan Back   Robert Grover   Sidney Udenfriend
George J. Brewer   Kurt Hirschhorn   Jonathan W. Uhr

Vol 1: **Erythrocyte Structure and Function,** George J. Brewer, *Editor*

Vol 2: **Preventability of Perinatal Injury,** Karlis Adamsons and Howard A. Fox, *Editors*

Vol 3: **Infections of the Fetus and the Newborn Infant,** Saul Krugman and Anne A. Gershon, *Editors*

Vol 4: **Conflicts in Childhood Cancer: An Evaluation of Current Management,** Lucius F. Sinks and John O. Godden, *Editors*

Vol 5: **Trace Components of Plasma: Isolation and Clinical Significance,** G.A. Jamieson and T.J. Greenwalt, *Editors*

Vol 6: **Prostatic Disease,** H. Marberger, H. Haschek, H.K.A. Schirmer, J.A.C. Colston, and E. Witkin, *Editors*

Vol 7: **Blood Pressure, Edema and Proteinuria in Pregnancy,** Emanuel A. Friedman, *Editor*

Vol 8: **Cell Surface Receptors,** Garth L. Nicolson, Michael A. Raftery, Martin Rodbell, and C. Fred Fox, *Editors*

Vol 9: **Membranes and Neoplasia: New Approaches and Strategies,** Vincent T. Marchesi, *Editor*

Vol 10: **Diabetes and Other Endocrine Disorders During Pregnancy and in the Newborn,** Maria I. New and Robert H. Fiser, *Editors*

Vol 11: **Clinical Uses of Frozen-Thawed Red Blood Cells,** John A. Griep, *Editor*

Vol 12: **Breast Cancer,** Albert C.W. Montague, Geary L. Stonesifer, Jr., and Edward F. Lewison, *Editors*

Vol 13: **The Granulocyte: Function and Clinical Utilization,** Tibor J. Greenwalt and G.A. Jamieson, *Editors*

Vol 14: **Zinc Metabolism: Current Aspects in Health and Disease,** George J. Brewer and Ananda S. Prasad, *Editors*

Vol 15: **Cellular Neurobiology,** Zach Hall, Regis Kelly, and C. Fred Fox, *Editors*

Vol 16: **HLA and Malignancy,** Gerald P. Murphy, *Editor*

Vol 17: **Cell Shape and Surface Architecture,** Jean Paul Revel, Ulf Henning, and C. Fred Fox, *Editors*

Vol 18: **Tay-Sachs Disease: Screening and Prevention,** Michael M. Kaback, *Editor*

Vol 19: **Blood Substitutes and Plasma Expanders,** G.A. Jamieson and T.J. Greenwalt, *Editors*

Vol 20: **Erythrocyte Membranes: Recent Clinical and Experimental Advances,** Walter C. Kruckeberg, John W. Eaton, and George J. Brewer, *Editors*

Vol 21: **The Red Cell,** George J. Brewer, *Editor*

Vol 22: **Molecular Aspects of Membrane Transport,** Dale Oxender and C. Fred Fox, *Editors*

Vol 23: **Cell Surface Carbohydrates and Biological Recognition,** Vincent T. Marchesi, Victor Ginsburg, Phillips W. Robbins, and C. Fred Fox, *Editors*

Vol 24: **Twin Research, Proceedings of the Second International Congress on Twin Studies,** Walter E. Nance, *Editor*
Published in 3 Volumes:
    Part A: **Psychology and Methodology**
    Part B: **Biology and Epidemiology**
    Part C: **Clinical Studies**

Vol 25: **Recent Advances in Clinical Oncology,** Tapan A. Hazra and Michael C. Beachley, *Editors*

Vol 26: **Origin and Natural History of Cell Lines,** Claudio Barigozzi, *Editor*

Vol 27: **Membrane Mechanisms of Drugs of Abuse,** Charles W. Sharp and Leo G. Abood, *Editors*

Vol 28: **The Blood Platelet in Transfusion Therapy,** G.A. Jamieson and Tibor J. Greenwalt, *Editors*

Vol 29: **Biomedical Applications of the Horseshoe Crab (Limulidae),** Elias Cohen, *Editor-in-Chief*

Vol 30: **Normal and Abnormal Red Cell Membranes,** Samuel E. Lux, Vincent T. Marchesi, and C. Fred Fox, *Editors*

Vol 31: **Transmembrane Signaling,** Mark Bitensky, R. John Collier, Donald F. Steiner, and C. Fred Fox, *Editors*

Vol 32: **Genetic Analysis of Common Diseases: Applications to Predictive Factors in Coronary Disease,** Charles F. Sing and Mark Skolnick, *Editors*

Vol 33: **Prostate Cancer and Hormone Receptors,** Gerald P. Murphy and Avery A. Sandberg, *Editors*

Vol 34: **The Management of Genetic Disorders,** Constantine J. Papadatos and Christos S. Bartsocas, *Editors*

Vol 35: **Antibiotics and Hospitals,** Carlo Grassi and Giuseppe Ostino, *Editors*

Vol 36: **Drug and Chemical Risks to the Fetus and Newborn,** Richard H. Schwarz and Sumner J. Yaffe, *Editors*

Vol 37: **Models for Prostate Cancer,** Gerald P. Murphy, *Editor*

Vol 38: **Ethics, Humanism, and Medicine,** Marc D. Basson, *Editor*

Vol 39: **Neurochemistry and Clinical Neurology,** Leontino Battistin, George Hashim, and Abel Lajtha, *Editors*

Vol 40: **Biological Recognition and Assembly,** David S. Eisenberg, James A. Lake, and C. Fred Fox, *Editors*

Vol 41: **Tumor Cell Surfaces and Malignancy,** Richard O. Hynes and C. Fred Fox, *Editors*

Vol 42: **Membranes, Receptors, and the Immune Response: 80 Years After Ehrlich's Side Chain Theory,** Edward P. Cohen and Heinz Köhler, *Editors*

Vol 43: **Immunobiology of the Erythrocyte,** S. Gerald Sandler, Jacob Nusbacher, and Moses S. Schanfield, *Editors*

Vol 44: **Perinatal Medicine Today,** Bruce K. Young, *Editor*

Vol 45: **Mammalian Genetics and Cancer: The Jackson Laboratory Fiftieth Anniversary Symposium,** Elizabeth S. Russell, *Editor*

Vol 46: **Etiology of Cleft Lip and Cleft Palate,** Michael Melnick, David Bixler, and Edward D. Shields, *Editors*

Vol 47: **New Developments With Human and Veterinary Vaccines,** A. Mizrahi, I. Hertman, M.A. Klingberg, and A. Kohn, *Editors*

Vol 48: **Cloning of Human Tumor Stem Cells,** Sydney E. Salmon, *Editor*

Vol 49: **Myelin: Chemistry and Biology,** George A. Hashim, *Editor*

Vol 50: **Rights and Responsibilities in Modern Medicine: The Second Volume in a Series on Ethics, Humanism, and Medicine,** Marc D. Basson, *Editor*

Vol 51: **The Function of Red Blood Cells: Erythrocyte Pathobiology,** Donald F. H. Wallach, *Editor*

Vol 52: **Conduction Velocity Distributions: A Population Approach to Electrophysiology of Nerve,** Leslie J. Dorfman, Kenneth L. Cummins, and Larry J. Leifer, *Editors*